Lifespan Processes

The Normal Events

John O. Towler, Ph.D.
Professor of Psychology
Renison College
University of Waterloo

160 Gould Street
Needham Heights, MA 02194

Printed in the United States of America

10 9 8 7 6 5 4 3 2 1

ISBN 0–536–58383–8
BA 7829

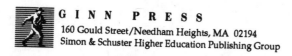

G I N N   P R E S S
160 Gould Street/Needham Heights, MA 02194
Simon & Schuster Higher Education Publishing Group

Contents

chapter 1

Getting a Framework
for the Lifespan

*Life is what happens to us while we
are making other plans.*

—Thomas La Mance

1. Introduction

This is really the preface, but I put it here because few people
actually read a preface unless they think they are going to be
acknowledged in it. I want to explain something about the book, its
style and where to get more information. I've approached the
topics as if I'm talking directly to you. Consequently, you'll find the
tone more conversational than some books and I'll share some of
my thoughts and experiences with you while asking you to think
about your ideas and the things that have happened to you.

The book will be much easier to read and more enjoyable this
way. I haven't put copious footnotes or references in the text because
I think they often interrupt the flow of information and distract the
reader from the points that are being made. However, I have given
you many sources where you can get more information on any topic
that interests you. I've simply listed these at the end of each chapter.

This material is so topical that new articles and books are
appearing every day. Don't forget to ask your friendly reference
librarian to help you locate these and additional materials. Every

academic library and many of the public ones will enable you to search for information using a computer. Even articles are now listed on CD ROMs. As useful as this book will be, your library will truly provide you with the keys to the kingdom if you are looking for more information.

One of the most difficult things about studying the entire life cycle is that of getting some perspective on it. How can anybody get an accurate view of all the things that may or may not happen over a lifespan? Part of the problem is that we have researched and learned about life in a pretty piecemeal fashion. It's natural to study what we are most interested in and the lifespan has been no exception. When our population was growing rapidly and more and more children were appearing, we concentrated on studying about children. As these children grew into adolescents, we turned our attention to this group and researched the development of adolescents. More recently as our population ages and the size of our elderly population grows, we have been turning our attention to the older adult. Now that we have become a nation of middle aged people, there are more of us who are more interested in our development so we are studying the young and middle aged adult.

Over the years we have learned a great deal about human development. We also know a considerable amount about the kinds of things that happen to people, how they react, what leads to the sort of problems that people can't handle on their own and even what type of issues and concerns most of us can expect to encounter. When we put it all together, this information can help us understand ourselves and others and prepare us for some of the things that can happen to us.

Now, what about the issue of how to fit all this into a manageable framework? The answer lies in knowing what to expect at each age and having some sort of system for putting it all together. This is where theories come in. It has been said that there is nothing as practical as a good theory and this will certainly be true here. We're not going to rely on many of them, but the ones that we will be looking at are the ones that you'll find most helpful in gaining a perspective on life. But I have to warn you. None of these theories is completely satisfactory. That is, no one of them gives us all the answers for the whole life cycle. But put together they give us a framework for our growing knowledge about people and how they change and develop.

2. Understanding the Theories

Before we get into these useful theories, there are some terms you will need to know and some points about the theories' strengths and weaknesses that you must keep in mind. Let's start with the idea of ages and stages. Most lifespan researchers such as *Erikson, Havighurst, Levinson, Neugarten, Gould* and *Vaillant* talk about stages (or passages, seasons or phases) that occur at different times in the lifespan. However, the stages overlap and are not consistently related to specific ages. In addition, the various researchers mean different things when they use the term stages. It may mean a transition, a crisis, an expectable event, a period of stability, a rite of passage or something else. The point is, we have been rather unsuccessful at identifying the stages that people go through, or even the events that happen to most people. We certainly cannot predict the ages when these events will occur. For example, you must not assume that everyone goes through the stages of getting married, having children and becoming part of a community. Some people do none of these things. Similarly, we cannot expect that these events will or ought to occur at certain ages. Even those who do get married may not do so in their 20s. Many get married now in their 30s and people (not always couples) have children at any age even up to and past menopause.

Another problem that lifespan theorists have wrestled with is the sequence in which events occur and why they happen when they do. While we can't pin these things down to a neat age-stage relationship, there is no doubt that most people experience a similar set of events such as becoming independent, marrying, having children, starting a career, and searching for identity. The question is why does this happen? Erikson's psychological model of development covers eight stages in the lifecycle. His theory explains that at certain ages there are specific issues that must be dealt with successfully before one can move on to the next stage of development. For example, he says that at about the age of 2 or 3, children must learn to assert their autonomy and that if they don't, they will develop feelings of self doubt and shame which will interfere with their psychological development.

Neugarten's psychosocial model isn't tied to specific ages, but involves what she calls a social time clock. This involves the values of the society in which we live and our understanding of what is normally expected of us at certain ages. I married when I was 23 and all my friends were getting married at that age too. This was the normal age for us to get married at that time. Today however, my children and their generation expect to get married much later, in their late 20s and early 30s. Society and our expectations have changed over the years.

Levinson's theory involves what he calls life structures. These are three points to remember about these common patterns of normal development. 1) They are dependent upon the world you are living in at the time (like Neugarten's social clock). 2)They involve the inner aspects of your life. This is like Erikson's idea of psychosocial development. 3) They include your degree of involvement in the world around you. This refers to your roles and relationships with others.

Then there is the whole question of what kinds of developmental tasks are associated with different periods of life. Havighurst is the best known researcher in this area. He identifies lists of tasks that we normally expect to develop at certain ages. For example he says that the normal development tasks of early adulthood are:

- getting started in an occupation
- selecting a mate
- learning to live with a partner
- starting a family

- rearing children
- taking on civic responsibility
- finding a congenial social group

If all of these sound somewhat similar, sensible, and interconnected, you are quite right. This is what makes it all rather confusing if you are trying to come up with a definitive answer to what life is all about. The best you can do is to take what makes the most sense to you from each of the theorists. Avoid falling onto the trap of assuming that we actually know what is normal for anyone at any given age, or thinking that we can predict what will or ought to occur at a specific age or time in our lives. The best way to make use of the theories is to treat them like a set of tools which can help you comprehend life. Just as you may need more than one kind of tool to do a job, you may need to select one or more of these theories to enable you to understand people and their development.

Life is not a problem to be solved but a reality to be experienced.

—Soren Kierkegaard

---

3. The Life Cycle According to Erik Erikson

Erikson was one of the first people to develop a theory that covered the complete lifespan. His eight stages of life begin at birth and end at death. Before we get to the theory itself, it is important to know a little about Erikson and the assumptions which underlie his work. You'll likely see some influence from Freud in Erikson's theory and it is true that Erikson accepts many of Freud's basic principles. He also believes that we have conscious and unconscious drives and that all children in all cultures go through the sequence of stages he outlines.

His theory is epigenetic. This term comes from the Latin epi and genesis meaning upon emergence. Erikson's point is that anything that grows has a predetermined pattern. Think of a flower. As each part grows, it appears at a specific time of ascendancy until all of the parts have developed to form a complete and properly functioning plant. Roots form then stems, then leaves, then flowers, then seeds, etc. He has applied the same idea to people and says that certain things will and should develop first, to be followed by others in a set sequence.

There are many detailed explanations of Erikson's theory and I'm not going to contribute another one here. But I do want to give you some examples of how it works, to demonstrate how you can use it to understand people and to explain why people may be acting like they are. Each stage consists of a turning point with two possible and opposing outcomes. One is positive and leads to future growth while the other outcome is negative and will interfere with development and may lead to maladjustment. I think that one of the most interesting things about this theory is that it explains how we develop important lasting outcomes which Erikson calls psychosocial strengths. These are shown in the last column of the chart below.

Stage One

This stage covers the first year of life. During this time, the infant must resolve the first psychosocial crisis of **Trust versus Mistrust**. If the child does so satisfactorily and learns to trust the world, this leads to the development of the ability of **Hope.** Think of it this way; baby Bruce comes home from the hospital; he is hungry and wet, and begins to cry. Upon hearing the cry, Bruce's mother comes to him, picks him up, feeds and gives him a hug and a kiss. Baby Bruce finds that each time he needs something, this wonderful creature called mother, appears and offers room service and love. Thus baby Bruce learns to trust his world and the people in it. Contrast this with baby Bonnie's experience. When she cries, her mother may or may nor come and may or may not feed, change,

Erik Erikson's Eight Stage Theory of the Lifespan

Stage	Age	Developmental Task	Psychosocial Strength
1	0–1	Trust vs. Mistrust	Hope
2	1–3	Autonomy vs. shame, doubt	Self control and will power
3	4–5	Initiative vs. guilt	Direction and purpose
4	6–12	Industry vs. inferiority	Competence
5	12–late teens	Identity vs. role confusion	Fidelity
6	early adulthood	Intimacy vs. isolation	Affiliation and love
7	middle adulthood	Generativity vs. Stagnation	Care
8	old age	Ego integrity vs. despair	Wisdom

and comfort her. This poor mom may be ill or on drugs, but whatever the reason she simply doesn't respond to baby Bonnie consistently or properly. Bonnie may learn that she cannot trust her world or some of the people in it.

Trust does lead to the capacity for hope. If we cannot or do not trust our world and the people in it, there is little reason for hope. Hope is essential in our society and most of us have learned to trust and hope. None of us for instance could possibly drive down the road if we didn't trust the other drivers to stay on their side of the road and to stop when the red lights are against them. An absence of hope would cripple us severely.

Stage Two

This stage covers the early childhood period which Erikson identifies as the second and third years of life. The Psychosocial crisis to be resolved now is that of **Autonomy versus Shame or Doubt**. During this stage, children are learning "right" from "wrong" and beginning to exercise self control. If we allow children to do things for themselves, they develop a feeling of **Autonomy**. But if we prevent them from doing things or criticize their results, they may feel ashamed of what they have done and learn to doubt their own abilities. Take for example the child who is learning to dress himself. Shirts are hard things to button when you are only two or three and shoe laces are even worse. Yet when most mothers and fathers try to help with these tasks they hear, "I can do it myself!" The results may not be what you expect and there may be the odd button left undone, but if the parents insist on doing it or tell the child that it is not correct, it can lead to an interference with the development of autonomy and a feeling of doubt or shame. If this crisis is resolved satisfactorily, the foundation for will power is formed. Will power for Erikson, means a sense of self-control without the loss of self esteem.

Stage Three

This is the play age of ages four and five and the crisis to be confronted is that of **Initiative versus Guilt.** It is natural for children to want to try things, to play with new toys, try out new games, associate with new people, etc. If we allow this to occur, Erikson says we are strengthening the drive towards initiative, but if we tell children that they are bad for having done these things, we are making them feel guilty for what they have done. In this case the psychosocial strength is that of **purpose.** This is the courage to take the initiative and do things without being paralyzed by guilt and the fear that one will be punished.

It's often hard to keep this in mind when children show their initiative in some ways. Consider what happens when children are given their first tricycle. We admonish them to not cross the road and to stay on the sidewalk. But the minute our backs are turned the child decides that it is time to ride around the block. The next time the parent looks out, their child has disappeared. The longer the parents look and call for the child, the more worried they get. Soon their thoughts turn to fears of abductions or accidents with large trucks. When they finally catch up with their child who is pedaling merrily along enjoying this first set of wheels, the parents are frantic and chastise the child for causing them so much worry. This is when the child ought to reply, "But I was only showing my natural initiative.

If you keep on like this, you'll make me feel guilty for what I've done and I'll never develop a sense of purpose!"

Stage Four

This covers the school age period from about age six to eleven and the tasks are **Industry versus Inferiority,** leading to the strength of **Competence**. During this time, the school has a great influence on children and often the teacher's opinion is more important than the parent's. The school system teaches children that if they work and meet certain standards they will be considered industrious and will be rewarded. If however, they don't work and perform satisfactorily, we give them poor grades and negative messages and teach them that they are inferior. Children who do what society tells them they should, develop a feeling of competence and ability. Erikson says that this factor is essential as a basis for cooperative participation in our culture.

Stage Five

This is the best known of Erikson's stages. It involves the adolescent ages from twelve to eighteen. The crisis now is that of **Identity versus Role Confusion** and its successful resolution leads to the strength of **Fidelity**. Fidelity as it is used here has a rather special meaning. It refers to the ability to be loyal to people and ideas even when they may contradict our own value systems. It is normal for adolescents to search for their own identities and to experiment with many activities, people, and values along the way. Most people develop a clear sense of who and what they are after a few years, and those who do not are, according to Erikson, experiencing role confusion. A knowledge of who you are and the ability to be comfortable with this is dependent in part on knowing what your own values are and being comfortable with them. If your own values are unclear and you are easily influenced by other people's values, you will find it hard to maintain lasting relationships or accept other people whose values differ from your own.

Stage Six

The young adult period is a rather vague one. Erikson wasn't very precise about it other than to say that it begins at the time of courtship and lasts into middle age. During this time, one must resolve the crisis of **Intimacy versus Isolation.** A satisfactory resolution leads to the strength of **Love.** But love as it is used here, means the ability to love another person to the extent that one overlooks the normal antagonisms and difficulties that arise when two people live together.

Erikson says that at this stage the identity is consolidated. This allows a person to overlook and ignore the demands for self gratification where these might interfere with a loving relationship. In other words, a person can love another and make significant sacrifices in doing so. The down side of this stage is the danger of possible psychological isolation or the refusal to get close enough to anyone to permit intimacy. In other words, a person at this end of the scale cannot or will not take another person's feelings or needs into account and will strengthen his or her own position, feelings, demands, etc., to the point where the other person is made to feel inferior. It has been said that a successful marriage requires each partner to put more than just a 50% effort into the relationship. A person who is unable to do so would be in danger of moving toward psychological isolation in Erikson's terms.

Stage Seven

Here too, Erikson's ages are very vague and he simply says that this period covers middle age. In this case, the crisis to be resolved is that of **Generativity versus Stagnation.** The successful resolution leads to the psychosocial strength of **care.** Generativity for Erikson, means a concern for and a desire to establish and guide the next generation. This needn't mean simply your children, it can also apply to younger workers in your firm or people in your community. This is the time in life, Erikson says, when we have a desire to return something to others and our community.

Generativity is a driving force in all healthy human organizations but if we don't reach out to others, a sense of stagnation and boredom may result. Care is a broad concept that refers to a concern for others and a continuation of the desire to look after other people rather than putting oneself first at all times.

Stage Eight

Integrity versus Despair. As you have probably anticipated by now, this stage is said to apply to the broad (and poorly defined) period of old age. A successful resolution leads to the psychosocial strength of **Wisdom.** The easiest way to understand this stage is to think of a person who, at the end of their life, looks back and considers what sort of life it has been. A fully developed person may say, "I think my life has been pretty good overall. Sure, there were things that I wish hadn't happened, but there were a lot of really wonderful things too and I wouldn't mind doing it all over again." A less developed person may say, "I hated my life. It was a disaster. The good times were few and far between and I'd never want to live it again." The first person has achieved some sort of satisfaction and closure about his or her existence and has accumulated some sort of knowledge and understanding about life, while the second person has learned very little and has a feeling of unhappiness and despair. People who have reached integrity, emotionally integrate their lives and past experience with the present and remain interested in the world around them. People who fail to achieve this feeling are left with a fear of death, a dissatisfaction about their lives and little understanding about what life has been all about. In Erikson's terminology, wisdom is a detached but active concern for life even though one recognizes that one's death is approaching.

One final but very important point before we leave my friend Erik. Even though he says that we pass through these stages in a set sequence and that these are normally encountered at certain ages, he also says that one can go through them again and again. Take the first stage of Trust versus Mistrust for example. Every time we establish a new relationship, join a new organization, attend a new school, live in a new country, etc., we have to re-learn who and what to trust. This is normal and natural. Erikson's point remains valid. How we resolve the issue will color our future development in that situation. Similarly, we go through many identity crises over the lifespan. Every time our roles change, we must figure out who we are now and how we should act. In other words, Erikson's theory is a useful way to look at what happens to us and how we react and grow over a very long period of time.

My grandfather always said that living is like licking honey off a thorn.

—Louis Adamic

---

4. Where Does This Leave Us?

Now that we have looked at a few of the most useful theories where do we go next and how can you actually use these ideas? Where we go next is easy, especially for me since I'm putting this together. I'm going to take you through the lifespan chronologically starting with childhood and ending up in old age, but I'm not just approaching it in the traditional manner of developmental psychology. I also want to help you understand how people cope with life, how they respond to problems, what happens when they find themselves in a crisis, and how they can be helped. I'll end the book with an interesting and provocative chapter on change, how it affects us and what we can anticipate in the way of changes in the future.

Regarding the question of how can you use these ideas, my students have found that the best way to understand and remember these concepts is to try to apply them. Luckily you have a ready-made experimental laboratory at your fingertips. Simply look around you and see if what you are reading helps you understand any of the people with whom you come into contact. Take Erikson for example. What stage are you at now? Which crises have you resolved and in which direction? Have you had to go through some more than once? What about your friends and parents? Where are they in this scheme. Most people find that the theories can be applied and that they make sense, but don't be alarmed if they don't fit you or your subjects exactly. After all, they are only theories.

> *The course of life is unpredictable . . . no one can write his autobiography in advance.*
>
> —Abraham Joshua Heschel

5. If You Want More Information

At the end of each chapter I will give you a list of the major references I have used for that section. I haven't put in every possible reference work you could possibly want, only a selection of the ones that you will find most useful. I've also tried to pick references that you will be able to find easily and read with the greatest understanding. There will certainly be many more books and articles on these topics, but the ones I'll list are the best ones with which to start.

References

Brim, O. G. Jr., and Kagan. *Constancy and Change in Human Development.* Cambridge: Harvard University Press. 1980.

Erikson, E. H. *Identity: Youth and Crisis.* New York: W. W. Norton. 1968.

Gould, R. L. *Transformations: Growth and Charge in Adult Life.* New York: Simon & Schuster. 1978.

Havinghurst, R. J. *Developmental Tasks and Education.* New York: McKay. 1972.

Lacy, W. B., and J. Hendricks. "Developmental Models and Adult Life: Myth or Reality." *International Journal of Aging and Human Development.* 112. 1980.

Levinson, D. J., C. N. Barrow, E. B. Klein, M. H. Levinson, and B. McKee, *The Seasons of Man's Life.* New York: A. A. Knopf. 1978.

Neugarten, B. L. "Time, Age, and the Life Cycles." *American Journal of Psychiatry. 136*7. 1979. p. 887–894.

Vaillant, G. E. *Adaptation to Life.* Boston: Little Brown. 1977.

chapter 2

Childhood and the Keys to Normal Development

A characteristic of the normal child is he doesn't act that way very often.

—Franklin P. Jones

---

1. The Developmental Tasks

Development is rapid in this period and there are many, many changes taking place in a relatively short period of time. Some of the major tasks to be completed in infancy are:

- learning to take solid foods
- learning to walk
- learning to talk
- learning to use the toilet
- learning sexual differences and personal modesty
- getting ready to read
- learning to distinguish between right and wrong
- developing a conscience

The developmental tasks of middle and late childhood include:

- learning physical skills needed for games
- building a wholesome attitude about oneself

- learning to get along with age-mates
- developing appropriate sex role behaviors
- developing fundamental reading, writing and numerical skills
- learning the concepts necessary for everyday living
- developing a more refined conscience, a sense of morality and personal values
- developing healthy attitudes towards people, groups, cultures and institutions
- achieving some personal degree of independence and control

2. How Has our Knowledge of Child Development Changed?

When we first began to study children and their development, we tended to focus on the physical and cognitive elements and we took a pretty mechanistic approach to the whole area. That is, we observed them and how they changed, what they did, how they developed and how they grew. However, there has been a revolutionary change in our understanding of children in the past 20 years and we have shifted away from the way we used to study them. Now we concentrate more on their cognitive and emotional development and the results of their interactions with their world. We also have come to realize that we have not paid enough attention to the issues of temperament, problem solving, creativity, social interaction abilities and the normal stresses involved in childhood.

One of the greatest influence in how we look at children was Jean Piaget, the Swiss psychologist who taught us so much about children's thought processes and their mental and moral capabilities. However, we are realizing now that his age-stage relationships aren't as accurate or as all encompassing as we first believed. Piaget's theory is comprehensive and complex and I'm not going to go into it in any detail here. Besides, it would seem most inappropriate since I've just told you that we no longer accept it the way we used to. However, you may recall that he postulated that child development was a matter of proceeding through a series of separate, age-related stages. He said that these stages and the steps in them were common to all children and that they all went through them in the same sequence. But over the years we have discovered more and more inconsistencies in Piaget's theories. For example, we now know that memory ability develops very rapidly up to about age five and then slows down through middle childhood and adolescence. Those who have studied it have discovered that this ability is dependent on learning how and when to remember and that children can be taught how to do this at a very young age. We've also learned that the development of problem solving abilities is not exactly the way Piaget explained it. Yes, if left to their own devices, children do tend to follow Piaget's stages of cognitive development and pass through concrete thinking to reach abstract hypothetical thought in what he called the stage of formal operations. But here too we have found that while problem solving improves naturally with age, a great deal of the improvement can be attributed to learning. For example, researchers at the University of Waterloo in Canada have found that children can be taught the importance of taking a systematic approach to solving a problem. They found that children who were poor at problem solving weren't so much delayed developmentally as they were simply impulsive and leaped to conclusions without thinking so that their conclusions were often wrong. However, they can be taught how to solve problems much earlier than Piaget suggested and the quality of their solutions is higher than we initially expected.

A similar thing has taken place concerning creativity. Now as every mother knows, all children are very imaginative and creative, at least when they are very young. Unfortunately, this seems to peak at about the time the child enters school where they learn that there is one right answer to certain questions, that there are right and wrong ways to do things and that it is now considered inappropriate to color grass pink and clouds green. In other words, our socializing process seems to constrict their natural creativity. But here again, we now know that progressive school programs and creativity training can enable children to keep and further develop their creative abilities.

The learning of social skills is another area where we have learned not only how children develop, but we can see ways to enhance this development. In essence we have discovered that becoming socially adept is a matter of learning the appropriate behaviours, and the appropriate scripts for given situations. It's a little like learning manners. If no one ever taught you to eat with your mouth closed, you would still be chewing away in an infantile, sloppy way. The same thing applies to learning how to interact in other aspects of our society. Children learn by imitation, instruction and experience. This has important implications for what kind of experiences we provide to children, what kind of models we present to them and what if anything we actually teach them about how to interact with society.

We have also come to realize that childhood isn't always the warm, peaceful period we think it is. Children experience a significant amount of stress in their daily lives, probably more than most of us are aware of. Like most other things, much of this is normal and most of us live through it and manage to cope and survive quite well. But if we are trying to get a better understanding of children and their development, it is important for us to know more about childhood stress, its causes and how to help children deal with it.

The outcome of all these changes in our thinking about how children develop is that we have come to realize that growing up is much more complex than we thought and that we cannot accurately predict its outcomes. We now know that a child's developmental competencies depend to a much larger extent on context, situation and experiences. Children are learning concepts and developing abilities that we once thought impossible at certain ages. We also know that age is not as important as what children are taught, how they are taught, how they are raised and cared for and the kind of homes and families in which they are raised. Of course this all has far reaching implications for families and educational systems. Unfortunately, there is a catch 22 problem here. While we want to help our children develop as fully as possible, there is a very real danger that we are propelling our children forward into an adult world too quickly. Authors such as Elkind and Postman have warned us that childhood is in danger of disappearing and that our children are growing up too fast and are being asked to become part of the adult world too soon.

> *If a child lives with approval, he learns to live with himself.*
>
> —Dorothy Law Nolte

3. Attachment, Competence and the Implications for Future Development

It is well known that mothers and their babies form a close and long lasting bond very soon after the baby is born. There is mounting evidence that this bonding is an essential element in child development and that it is the basis for a wide variety of future competencies. It is now very clear that a baby's early experiences affect the development of attitudes, fears, and expectations that will influence how the baby behaves as a child and even as an adult.

The concept we will be talking about here is that of attachment. Attachment is the special intimacy and closeness that forms between a baby and its primary caregiver (this may or may not be the baby's mother) during the first year of life. Babies like to feel comfortable, secure, and loved and they normally get these feelings from the person who cares for them. Babies who are progressing normally and in a healthy manner are developing strong attachments with their caregivers. This attachment allows the baby to explore its environment and to achieve a kind of comfortable mastery over it. The kinds of attachment, how they develop, and their immediate and long term effects have been studied by many people, but one of the best known researchers is Mary Ainsworth. Ainsworth uses a three level system to explain attachment.

The Three Types of Attachment	
Securely Attached	*Insecurely Attached*
1. Securely Attached	1. Ambivalent Attached
	2. Avoidantly Attached

There is the securely attached and two kinds of anxious attachment—ambivalent and avoidant. But before we get to this, I'd better explain how researchers study attachment in babies. They do it by means of an experiment known as the strange situation. Here's how it works. The caregiver (let's call her the mother in this case) and her baby come into an unfamiliar room in which there are some toys and a stranger. *Securely* attached children will leave their mother's side and begin to play with the toys. After a few minutes, they may warm up to the stranger who has been talking with their mother. Next the mother leaves the room. At this point, the baby feels some stress and almost all babies show some signs of this. They may fret, become upset or stop playing for a time. When the mother returns, the baby usually goes to her, makes physical contact, gets comforted, and then resumes playing.

Anxiously attached children respond in quite a different way. An *ambivalently* attached baby in the same strange situation experiment responds as follows. These babies do not do as much exploring of the room and the toys as the securely attached babies and they stick very close to their mothers. They do not warm up to the stranger while the mother is present and become very upset when the mother leaves the room. They are very wary of the stranger and continue to show acute discomfort and stop playing while the mother is absent. But even when the mother returns, they cannot settle down and are ambivalent in their attitudes to their mother and the room. They mix resistance to their mother with seeking contact with her. They may push her away, hit at her, knock the toys away, and, in general, show their discontent with the situation and their mother. Naturally this interferes greatly with their ability to explore the room and enjoy the toys.

The second category of anxiously attached babies, the *avoidant* babies *appear* to be well behaved and well adjusted but don't be fooled. This seemingly good behaviour is a symptom of something that has gone very wrong. These babies don't seem to care whether the mother is there or not in that they separate readily from them and do not seek contact. They are not wary of the stranger and do not seem to be upset when the mother leaves. Even when she returns, the baby does not seek renewed contact and may actually ignore her. If she approaches, they purposely try to avoid her. It's as if the babies have decided that they will protect themselves from any hurt by becoming purposely aloof from everyone. The effects of these kinds of attachment are not only interesting, they are extremely important, long lasting and quite disturbing in their implication for the development of future competencies. While not all researchers are in complete agreement about this, there is a growing body of evidence that how a baby becomes attached and what kind of attachment is obtained will have effects that last well into the childhood years and perhaps beyond. Consider these findings. Babies who were studied at 18 months were found to exhibit behaviours that varied according to their type of attachment. Securely attached children were more enthusiastic and persistent and demonstrated more positive feelings than did anxiously attached children. The securely attached also showed fewer negative emotions, were more compliant, had fewer temper tantrums and were less oppositional with their mothers and showed less aggression than their anxiously attached counterparts. Interestingly enough, these studies also show that there is a difference between the mothers of anxiously and securely attached children with the latter being more supportive and interested in their children.

At the age of 2 years the differences not only persist but are more visible. Insecurely attached children are frustrated easily and tend to be whinny, lack self-reliance, and show little interest in solving problems. By age 3 these children are characterized as problem children by their teachers and demonstrate poor peer relationships and little resilience. By the time they reach the age of 6 they demonstrate hopelessness when threatened with separation. Other studies have found that avoidant children are less able to involve themselves in creative fantasy and that when they play with other children, they tend to become involved in irresolvable conflicts. In addition, they seem to be more prone to victimize other avoidant children, are sullen, oppositional, and unwilling to seek help when they need it.

Researchers have also found that a certain type of personality seems to be associated with anxiously and securely attached children. The securely attached children are significantly more sympathetic towards other children, are more likely to be peer leaders; they attract the attention of other children, suggest more activities and are more self directed. On the other hand, insecurely attached children have been found to be significantly more hesitant with other children, wary about engaging in activities, incurious about new things, socially withdrawn, and avoidant of excitement and activities. Research with the strange situation experiment has time and again produced results that indicate that about two thirds of our middle class children are securely attached and about one third fall into the two insecurely attached categories. Not enough research has been done to be able to comment authoritatively yet on what proportions we might find in lower class families or the children of broken or dysfunctional families.

What does it all mean? If nothing else, it has fueled a great controversy about day care and the effects on children. Those who believe strongly in the attachment findings feel that full time day care during the first year is a very dangerous thing and that it should not be left to just anyone. Clearly there is reason to believe that the first few years of life are extremely important for the healthy development of the child and that the lessons they learn during this period will have a long term effect on their ability to make their way in the world, adapt and get along with people. We don't know whether these effects last forever or whether they can be reversed, but it seems abundantly clear that these effects do exist and that they have the potential for causing problems later on in life. The answers aren't all in yet, but coupled with what we now know about the long lasting effects of family disintegration on children and the problems this is creating for our society, it seems reasonable to assume that the two issues are tied together.

Children need love, especially when they do not deserve it.

—Harold S. Hulbert

---

4. Do Children Experience Stress?

In a word, yes. Childhood isn't the carefree time we'd like to think of it as. Despite what the Disney channel and other media sources would like to have us believe, childhood for most children is a time of constant change, adjustment, anxiety, and stress. Now that's not to say that it isn't enjoyable and most of us look back quite naturally on our childhood with happy memories and a generally good feeling. My point is that as adults we have forgotten just how stressful childhood can be.

Like it or not, stress seems to be a normal part of our world and it is a factor in everyone's life, even children. When you stop to think about it, there are a whole host of things that can produce stress in children. I'm going to outline most of them here to give you an overview of the situation. The section of childhood fears which follows will give you more details about the topic and if you are looking for what to do about it, you'll find the answers in chapter eight.

The things that cause stress for children

- physical illness
- pain
- concentration
- failure at school, a task, on a team, etc.
- going to the dentist
- going to the hospital
- coming home alone after school
- being teased
- feeling unloved
- living in a dangerous neighborhood
- violence on television
- physical or mental abuse
- a dysfunctional family
- too much stimulation
- a death in the family
- divorce and separation

The list can go on and on and you begin to wonder whether any children escape these stresses. Whatever the cause, stress affects children in fairly similar ways. Depending on their age and experience, they may become shy and withdrawn, or boisterous and aggressive. They may seem terrified or become antisocial. If they are very young, they may regress to bedwetting and thumbsucking. Stress in children is hard to study because the children respond in so many different ways, and because it is difficult to separate the stressors from all the other things that are going on in the child's life at the same time. Nevertheless, we do know that male children are more susceptible to stress than female children, or at least they show more symptoms of stress. We also know some of the major causes of stress. Much of this may seem like plain common sense, but the point is that we tend to dismiss stress in children as something that either doesn't happen or as something that is of little importance. It may not be important to the adults who have other things on their minds, but it is certainly very important to the children who are experiencing stress.

Here are some of the stressors that we know affect children. *Crowded, crime ridden neighborhoods.* This is becoming a "normal" state of affairs in our cities and children who live in these conditions may fear for their own safety, for their friends and they may not have the privacy and space that they they need to play . There is a cultural factor at work here though, since we know that children raised in very densely populated cities like Hong Kong don't feel the same amount of stress as our inner city children. *Poverty* is another major stressor for far too many children. Poverty, low socioeconomic status, parental job loss, and all the negative things that go along with these factors often result in heightened tensions in the home and increases in mental and physical abuse. The stressors that are harder for us to see as adults are the ones that we never seem to think of as bothering children. These include such things as natural disasters and the fear of war. The recent earthquakes in California, the 1993 winter "storm of the century" that hit the American sun belt just as the school children and their families were heading to Disneyland are just two of the natural occurrences that cause anybody stress and affect children in particular. But it doesn't end with the things that actually touch us. In this day of constant news coverage and instant reporting, things like war, terrorism, starvation, and civil insurrection are brought into the home on a regular basis. All of these things were always terrible, but at least in my childhood they weren't as real, as near, or put before me on a constant basis. No wonder children fear these things. Adults do too.

But even in the regular scheme of things in a normal family there are occurrences that we adults think of as simply a commonplace part of life, yet these events are highly disturbing to children. These include the birth of a sibling, the death of a pet, a sick parent, a dying grandparent, etc. Each of these can be a major source of fear and concern for children *even if they aren't happening!* In other words, children allow their imaginations to lead them into worries that may not take place. As an only child, I remember worrying about who would take care of me if my parents died. As I recall, I went over the list of all my parent's relatives and friends and terrified myself with a series of horrendous "what if" scenarios. My students tell me they have also engaged in this kind of childhood worry.

However, some of the things that children fear the most, actually do happen. Two of the most serious are the death of a parent and the divorce of one's parents. Both of these things can and often do have long lasting effects on children, even adult children. It's all too easy while we are caught up at these times in our own emotions to forget that the children are suffering significant amounts of stress too.

Now lest you find this all too stressful yourself, remember that children are surprisingly resilient and that people, children included, survive these events and live to tell about it. However, it would be a better world if we were more aware of childrens' stresses, were able to shield them from the things that worry them or to help them cope when they are beset by such worries.

By the time the youngest children have learned to keep the house tidy, the oldest grandchildren are on hand to tear it to pieces.

—Christopher Morley

---

5. The Sources and Kinds of Child Stress

One of the great stress researchers, Hans Selye, identified eleven major causes of stress in adults. Yes, I know that we are talking about stress in children, but the relationship is a good one and I'll make the connection in a minute. Here are the eleven stressors that

Selye discovered. You'll see that there are counterparts for each of them for children.

---

1. Job
2. Human Relations
3. Climate
4. Crowding
5. Boredom
6. Loneliness
7. Captivity
8. Relocation
9. Urbanization
10. Catastrophe
11. Anxiety

There probably isn't an adult among us who would quarrel with that list, but it is surprisingly applicable to children too. Let's take a look at each one and see how it applies to children.

1. Job—For children, this is school and the six hours that they spend there every day are filled with problems, pressures, pleasures, and interactions with playmates, teachers, authority, bullies, and new things to learn. A child's survival and self image is on the line every day.

2. Human relations—Here too children must cope with many people both at school and at home every day. But the thing to remember here is that children are very intense in their relationships and that they are never indifferent. Minor slights are seen as major events and friendships shift daily and even hourly. Your best friend one minute can be a hateful enemy the next. A child's emotions range through love, hate, fear, delight, anger, and envy almost daily.

3. Climate—Selye means the physical weather climate and as every parent and teacher knows, children are dramatically affected by the weather. Rainy days seem to bring out the beast in children and they are louder, more uncontrollable, more prone to arguing and moping around than when the sun is shining.

4. Crowding—This seems to affect all species and there have been some great experiments with rats showing that when the cages become too crowded, the social order breaks down and aggression takes over. This really shouldn't be a surprise to us, but when we apply this to children's lives we see that they are often in crowded places either at home in high rises, crowded cities or at school where they spend their days in large groups, in overcrowded classrooms, and overcrowded schools.

5. Boredom—All too often this seems to be a normal state of affairs for children and every parent has heard the plaintive wail, "There's nothing to do!" As one gets older one learns not to say this because it invariably leads to the dreaded suggestion that you clean your room, take out the garbage, or cut the lawn. Nevertheless, children all too often turn to television to alleviate boredom and we now find that 40 hours a week of TV are not uncommon in the lives of most children. This is more time than they spend in school! Consequently, children expect to be bored, especially in school.

6. Loneliness—This is the hallmark of the adolescent's existence. It comes in part from a sense of not quite belonging. Older children who are moving away from parents to the peer group may find that they don't feel comfortable with either for years. Children like familiarity and security, but many times they find themselves in lonely situations. This is probably even more the case with latch key children who come home alone to empty houses. Not all of them are as self reliant as movies like "Home Alone" would have us believe.

7. Captivity—I think that one of the most dreadful things to experience would be that of being held captive as a hostage. Yet we

accept it as normal that all children live their lives in a sort of captivity where they have little if anything to say about the rules and regulations by which they must live. They have no control over whether they will attend school, what classes they will take, with whom they will live, where they will live, etc. As we'll see later, a lack of control is a key factor is stress and children have very little control.

8. Relocation—If this causes adults stress, it is a fact of life for children. They are relocated daily from class to class, lesson to lesson, and are forced to see relatives, attend events, and go places that their parents determine. This is the normal state of their world. It becomes much worse and more stressful when a parent gets a new job or there is a divorce. Then there are relocations to new homes, new relatives, new schools, new friends, etc.

9. Urbanization—This is a problem for both adults and children as they cope with the pressures and problems of living in urban centres. However, the children often feel it more keenly as they contend with where to ride their bikes, where to play an outdoor game, how to get close to nature, how best to travel to a friend's place and nowadays, how to protect oneself from molesters and abductors. Adults don't experience these pressures and are generally unaware of them in the child's world.

10. Catastrophe—For adults this means natural catastrophes like fire, flood, and war and all the ensuing dangers and disruptions they can bring. But catastrophe has an entirely different meaning for a child. For them, *everything* is a catastrophe! A friend who won't speak to you, a sick pet, a failed exam, a sarcastic teacher, an unhappy parent, or even leaving your lunch on the bus is a major catastrophe. Children seem to live constantly on the edge of disaster and to see their world in these terms.

11. Anxiety—As you'll see later, many adults are so stressed about one thing or another they have difficulty pinning the stress

down to any one factor. We say that they are suffering from free floating anxiety. Well, the same is true for children and anxiety is almost a normal state for them. They worry about who loves or likes them, whether they will succeed in school, be picked for a team or the school play, whether they are too fat or too thin, whether they will grow too much or too little, and a whole host of other things that enter their fertile, worrying minds.

When you look at all these factors it's easy to see that childhood isn't really the carefree time we assume it is. The point to remember here is that childhood stress is real and very worrisome for many children. However, you must also remember that it is normal, that there are ways to handle it, to help children cope with it, and that we all seem to survive childhood and mainly enjoy the process. We really are tough, resilient creatures aren't we?

---

*The modern child will answer you
back before you've said anything.*

—Laurence J. Peter

Selye wasn't the only person to study childhood fears, of course, and our friend Erik Erikson also had some interesting insights into the source of child stress. Interestingly enough, he too identified eleven basic fears.

1. Fear of Withdrawal of Support—Children naturally fear that other people whom they respect will withdraw their support, especially if they do something bad. Hence children may fear that a parent will withdraw support if they let them down by not performing or obeying their rules. Of course this is a major pressure in school where teachers regularly hand out good marks, approval, and encouragement to those who perform,

and withhold all of these from those who don't. But it can also apply to one's peer group who offer ridicule instead of support if one wears the wrong clothes, listens to the wrong music, or differs from the groups' values.

2. Fear of Suddenness—Initially, parents move slowly and quietly so they don't needlessly disturb their babies. But as the children grow the children are subjected to more and more sudden changes. It was OK to stay up late last night, but not tonight. At school the child's world is governed by bells and the clock and one must change classes, teachers, and rooms at specific times. The sudden changes also extend to major alterations which seem to be sprung on the children with little warning or consultation as when the parents decide to move to another house or city, or when the children are taken to grandmother for the day.

3. Fear of Noise—Most adults savour a quiet time by themselves, but when you stop to think about it, the child's world is an incredibly noisy one. The home can be very noisy with parents, siblings, the TV, and the stereo all competing to be heard over the washing machine, the telephone, and a myriad of other things. Somehow our world has become noisier and noisier and we have learned to accept it. All too often we perpetuate the noise at alarming levels as any parent who visits a rock concert will attest. Nevertheless, these noises and the levels we live with are all disturbing.

4. Fear of Being Manipulated—No one wants to be manipulated either physically or psychologically. Any parent who has gone through the experience of putting a child into a snowsuit will remember all too well how squirmy the child becomes and how every limb suddenly turns to rubber. Children seem to be at their worst when we are helping them get dressed in anything. We are always manipulating children. Schools manipulate children regularly with regulations from everything from dress codes to what one is allowed to do at any given moment of the

day. Parents too set up confining rules, many of which are created for the benefits of the parents, not the children. The insistence that one clean one's room is certainly more due to the fact that mother can't stand it than because junior can't abide it any longer.

5. Fear of Interruption of a Vital Activity—This is probably one of my favorites in the list because everything is a vital activity for children. That is, whatever they are doing at the time, (if they like it,) is an essential thing that simply must be done now. Reading a comic book, talking with a friend, skipping rope, playing ball, or simply sitting doing nothing is always more important than whatever someone else wants to have the child do at that particular moment. Yet the world of the child is such that we constantly interfere and interrupt them to have them do something else. This has an easily recognized link to the issue of being in control of one's own world.

6. Fear of Being Deprived of a Valuable Possession—Children are very possessive and love to hoard things, collect items and be surrounded by special things. The problem is that we adults fail to remember that we were like this and to recognize the importance of a child's valuable possessions. Partly this is because we have difficulty in recognizing what is and is not important to them. There's probably not a family around that hasn't come to grief because Billy's rock collection was thrown out or Susie's comic books were moved out of her room. I heard one father tell about how his four-year-old gave him a small box of bits and pieces to take to his office. He did so, and several weeks later threw it away only to be asked that night when he was going to bring back his child's box of treasures that had been entrusted to his safekeeping! In these days of increasing crime, children are very concerned that their things will be stolen and all too many of them have already had that experience. The memories of these events leave a lasting impression. If you doubt this, think back to the first important thing you had taken

from you. Everyone can recall this with amazing clarity and anger.

7. Fear of Restraint—All children hate to be held down and restrained. Yet they are constantly subject to all kinds of restraint, both physical and psychological. We are forever telling them what to do or not to do something. In school they must sit still for hours, something that is really quite unnatural for children. One study asked a group of high school students to select the one word from a list that best described their school. You won't be surprised to learn that the word most of them chose was "prison."

8. Fear of Having No Imposed Controls—Now you would think that after we have made this case that children are so hard done by with all the controls we impose, that the last thing they would want is more controls. Yet, this is exactly what children actually wish. It's one thing to have too many restrictions, but it's even worse to have none at all. Much of the difficulties children get into stem from their natural curiosity to test the limits to which they can go and just how firm their parents' and teacher's rules actually are. But the child with no restrictions or guidelines is filled with doubts, fears, and guilts. In a strange way, it is somehow comforting to know what one can and cannot do. A lack of controls often leads to unhappiness.

9. Fear of Being Exposed—No one, including children, wants to be examined, investigated, found out, and exposed to anyone. But this is also part of the normal work of the child. We ask "Did you clean your teeth? Are your hands washed? Did you do your homework?" and often we don't take the answer at face value, we check to see if the task was done at all or done properly. Constant inspection deprives people of dignity and children are no exception.

10. Fear of Remaining Small—Size is important in our society and we equate largeness with superior qualities. We think that big

stores are better than small ones, big cars more impressive than tiny ones, big movies superior to short, low budget ones, etc. Children quickly internalize these attitudes, but in their case, *everything* is bigger than they are. Consequently, they fear that they will not grow up, or up far enough. Often parents reinforce this fear. I remember a childhood friend whose parents were both very short. Naturally he too was on the short side. We both attended a "swim and gym" club at the local Y, but my poor friend was instructed by his mother to spend a good part of his time in the gym hanging from the flying rings in the hopes that it would stretch him out. As I recall, he did this faithfully, but it never offset the genes that he had inherited.

11. Fear of Being Left Alone—This fear relates back to the attachment issue and the natural fear that children have that their parents will die and they will be left behind. This fear is often strengthened when grandparents die. Today's latchkey children often have to deal with this fear on a daily basis.

Now that you know more about these fears, what can you do about it? First of all, you must realize that this is a normal state of affairs and the most exemplary parents and teachers cannot eliminate all these stresses no matter what they do. Secondly, you should realize that learning to confront and cope with these fears is an essential part of growing up. Nevertheless, you should understand that children do live with constant stress. You should become more aware of these stressors and their causes and try to eliminate the unnecessary ones. We'll get to the methods for dealing with stress and learning how to cope more effectively in chapter seven.

*Before I got married I had six theories
about bringing up children; now I
have six children and no theories.*

—John Wilmot, Earl of Rochester (1647–1680)

5. Where to Find More Information

Cowan, P. *Piaget with feeling.* New York: Holt, Rinehart & Winston. 1978.

Ginsburg, H., and S. Opper. *Piaget's Theory of Intellectual Development.* (2nd ed.) Englewood Cliffs, NJ: Prentice Hall. 1989.

Sroufe, L.A., and J. Fleeson. *Attachment and Construction of Relationships.* In W. Hartup and Z. Rubin (Eds.), *Relationships and Development.* Hillsdale, NJ: Erlbaum. 1986.

Whitee, B.L. *The First Three Years of Life.* New York: Prentice Hall. 1990.

Karen, R. "Becoming Attached." *Atlantic Monthly.* Feb., 1990. 35-70.

Miller, M. S. *Child-Stress! Understanding & Answering Stress Signals of Infants, Children & Teenagers.* Garden City, NY: Doubleday, 1982.

Piaget, J. "Development and Learning." *Journal of Research in Science Teaching.* 1964. p. 176–86.

Ranieri, R. F. "Helping Children Cope With Divorce." *Marriage and Family Living.* Apr., 1980. p. 18–21.

Zineister, K. "Growing up Scared." *Atlantic Monthly.* June, 1990. p. 49–66.

McCook, S. "When a Child Worries—How to Recognize and Relieve Childhood Stress." *Canadian Living.* 1987, 5, p. 101–4.

Youngs, B. B. *Stress in Children—Common Sense Advice on How to Spot and Deal With Stress in Children of All Ages.* New York: Arbor House. 1985.

Honig, A. S. "Stress and Coping in Children." *Young Children.* May, 1986.

Sroufe, L. A. "Attachment and the Roots of Competence." *Human Nature.* Oct., 1978.

Chance, P., and J. Fischman. "The Magic of Childhood." *Psychology Today.* May, 1987. p. 48.

chapter 3

The Adolescent Years

Heredity is what sets the parents of a teen-ager wondering about each other.

—Laurence J. Peter

---

1. Introduction

For some parents, even the term "adolescent" sends shivers down their spines. Usually this isn't because they think back with delight to their own adolescent, but because they shudder to think of what it must or will be like to raise their own teenagers. Like many other things, there is mixture of myth and truth in this. The adolescent years are certainly interesting to say the least, but they aren't necessarily the period of unbridled rebellion, stress, and turmoil that they have been made out to be. My objective in this chapter is to tell you the facts, to examine what normally happens and why, and to assist you to get not only a better understanding about what is or may be likely to happen, but a handle on what you can do to live comfortably with people at this interesting age.

2. The Developmental Tasks

There aren't as many developmental tasks at this age as there were for the rapidly growing and developing younger child, but the things that an adolescent must be able to do are much more complex or at least they seem that way because they nearly always involve other people. Some of the developmental tasks that have been identified are:

- achieving a personal identity
- building new relationships with one's peers
- becoming aware of one's own sexuality
- achieving a sex role
- coping with a growing and developing body
- becoming involved with the opposite sex
- becoming socially responsible
- separating from parents
- preparing for a future career
- preparing for marriage and family life
- acquiring ethics and a set of values

Just look over this list. Each of these tasks is a major undertaking and you would be hard pressed to help anybody learn everything that they need to know to be able to handle any one of these items. Somehow most adolescents get these things figured out quite satisfactorily, but it is no wonder that it takes some experimentation, that it doesn't happen overnight and that there will be mistakes and some difficulties along the way. That's life!

3. When Does Adulthood Begin?— The Adolescent Moratorium

How does one know when they are no longer a child? Can anybody tell by looking at a person that they are "adult"? This is one of the things that is very difficult, at least in our society. We seem to stretch the period of adolescence out for years and nobody including the adolescents has a definitive idea about when it begins or when it ends. A few years ago when I asked my students to give me the ages when adolescence begins and when one becomes an adult, they used to tell me that it started about age 12 and lasted until the end of the teenage years. Now when I ask them I get ranges from as early as 10 ("That's when my sister started dating."), or 11 ("That's when puberty begins for most girls now."), to the 20s ("When you finally get established and get a job."), or never ("Because some people never seem to grow up."). Think about it yourself. What would you say?

Whatever you think, it is certainly true that we have stretched the period we know as *adolescence* out over many years and it seems to be lasting longer and longer. It's as if we have put a moratorium on adolescence. Partly this is because people are staying in school longer, delaying getting married until later, and finding it harder to get established in some of the adult roles such as homeowner and having a career. The problem is that we have no easily observable markers to let us know when one stops being a child and when one enters the adult world.

However, there are cultures that have always had ceremonies or rituals that marked an individual's transition from the status of child to that of being an adult. These *rites of passage* were important and useful in that they let the child and others know just what they were. Wherever these rites existed, the always had several things in common.

First of all, they were public events that took place before the other members of the community. Secondly, they were set rituals which were used time and time again in a traditional manner. Thirdly, they marked the completion of some task that the child had performed. And lastly, the child was granted entrance to the adult world; was allowed to know things that only other adults knew and had to take on new responsibilities in keeping with the new adult status.

Now before you wish that we had such rites today, we'd better look at what some of these rites involved. In some primitive tribes the boys were removed from their parents, underwent ritual circumcision, and were sent into the forest to perform a feat of strength, to kill a certain beast, or to fast and experience hallucinations. Those who were able to complete the tasks were told the secrets of the tribe, instructed on their new adult responsibilities, perhaps marked with distinctive tattoos or other markings, dressed differently, and were then presented to the rest of the community. But after this, they were not allowed to return to live with their parents, but had to live with the other adults until they married. Girls too went through similar rites including circumcision and traditional marking and a change in clothing.

Now as strange as all this may sound, it did have the advantage of helping everyone understand their roles and just what stage they were at in life. We have nothing that is comparable to these rites and this is one of the reasons we and our adolescents are confused about whether they are adults or not. To be sure, we have some vestiges of these ceremonies, but they don't really fit the four criteria outlined above. Some of our modern "rites of passage" include such things as:

- the first communion
- a bar or bat mitzvah
- getting a driver's license
- losing one's virginity
- being able to legally vote, or drink

- graduating from high school (now university?)
- getting married
- being presented as a debutante

However, you can easily see that these rites fail to mark the entrance into the adult world. They occur at a wide range of ages, some only apply to one sex, some are private not public events, not everyone goes through them, some of them don't require the successful completion of anything except getting older, and none of them mark the time when the initiate learns adult secrets they didn't know before. In fact, when you consider the last point, the case can be made that there are very few if any things that children and adolescents don't know about life and the adults' world. Today's elementary school age child knows more about sex than I did when I was a teenager and very few of us ever learned these adult facts from our elders.

So where does this leave us? With the understanding that life as or with an adolescent is very different now than it used to be and we are all less sure about when one stops being a child and moves into the adult world for good.

It's hard for the modern generation to understand Thoreau, who lived beside a pond but didn't own water skis or a snorkel.

—Bill Vaughen

---

4. What Are the Normal Changes We Can Really Expect To See In Adolescence?

Here again, I'm not going to give you an exhaustive list of what happens or a short course on adolescence. There are many good books and courses that do that very well. What I want to do here is to give you a flavor of the kinds of things that are normal and to be expected during this phase. It is important to understand that going through adolescence is a normal crisis of life. People at this age are experiencing major changes in behaviour, physical shape and function, emotions and attitudes towards themselves and others. Intellectually, they have developed most of the capabilities they will need for the adult world, but they sometimes have difficulty applying them consistently. One day they can be sound reasoners and the next the emotional side takes over and they revert to being irrational children.

The major, most easily observed changes are due to puberty. This is starting earlier and earlier and we normally expect its onset at about 11. It is accompanied by a host of alterations not the lest of which is menstruation in girls and the growth of the penis and testes in boys. The signs that are most visible are the growth spurt in both sexes and the development of breasts and the widening of the hips in girls and the shoulders in boys. This can either be exciting and delightful and a source of pride or a frightening shameful thing. Often parents feed either of these attitudes consciously or unconsciously. One of the most annoying problems for boys is learning how to control this growing body and some may be very ungainly and awkward for a time. I remember our own sons at this age. For a few years we couldn't keep up to their growth and new pants only lasted a few months before they were too short and the sleeves in shirts seemed to shrink before our eyes. The weren't particularly awkward, but I recall them unexpectedly bumping into things (especially me) more than I was used to.

Of course the other change that drives parents crazy is the denigration of everything parental. Annoying as it may be, this too is normal and you can only strive to rise above it and feel sympathetic for the poor adolescents who are trying to assert their independence, determine their identities while denying their fears, and feelings of incompetence while being caught in a dilemma in which they are still dependent on and need the protection of their parents. Couple this with a hefty dose of bravado and a pseudo sophistication in which they claim to know everything about anything and you have a recipe for trouble. This is why, in the same breath, an adolescent may tell her parents that they are stupid and that they are not looking after her properly.

Adolescents also go through periods of mood swings, like to withdraw from the world and experiment with new bodies, new ideas, and creative urges. It's really quite an exciting time and at the end of it, the adolescent has integrated all of these experiences, formed a cohesive identity, developed an integrity of character and a sound value system. Learning to live with them as they go through this period may call for patience and understanding and the realization that it is normal for them and for parents to engage in a certain amount of yelling. At about the age of 14 our boys turned into flaming adolescents and they didn't rejoin the human race until they turned 16. However, everyone including the parents do survive this period. It is a normal and necessary part of growing up.

> *In case you're worried about what's going to become of the younger generation, it's going to grow up and start worrying about the younger generation.*
>
> —Roger Allen

5. Achieving An Identity

One of the major tasks during this period is that of determining one's identity, but just what is involved and how does one actually do this? Unfortunately, it's not as easy as it used to be. Years ago, we had a few basic reference points that told us and everyone else around us who we were. These included such things as ancestry, age, sex, occupation, religion, place of birth, where we lived, etc. Men worked and were fathers, women had children and worked in the home. Our communities were stable and homogeneous and everyone was quite clear about who and what they were.

Today, however, the world is a very different place and we can change some of the reference points that served as markers for our identity. We move from place to place, from job to job, and in and out of marriages. We change jobs, our religious and political orientations, our names and some now change their sex. Consequently, our identities are tied not only to the old reference points, but to more fluid ones tied more closely to things that are under our control. Today, we seem to have multiple roles and multiple identities. It's more accurate, though to say that our identities are more complex and that they are made up of a multiplicity of factors. In fact, the greater choices we have now, make it much harder for us to decide who we are and what we want to be. The old sex role stereotypes that said that women work at home and men work outside the home, at least guided us to some degree. Now that we are breaking these down and women are taking their places in executive suites and men are becoming more involved in the home, it is much harder to determine what we think we are supposed to be. In fact, the great number of choices that one has in a democracy and the prevailing attitude that one can be anything one sets out to be, means that people, especially young people are naturally confused about what they want to be, who they are, and who they should become. But a rush to find an identity can lead to over-identification in which we convince ourselves that we are very much like this or that group and that we must emulate them. This is really a defense against uncertainty and the uncomfortable feelings that go along with this state. Unfortunately, parents often contribute to this drive to associate with any identity when they demand that their teenagers figure out what they want to be and get on with the job. Anyone who has looked at a university or college calendar or a list of current occupations would realize that there is a bewildering array of choice just in the area of careers.

The people who seem to have the hardest time determining an identity are those who have trouble juggling multiple roles simultaneously. But who among us doesn't play many roles during the course of even one day. How many roles have you played today? You may have been parent, child, employee, student, researcher, cook, housekeeper, and chauffeur. But some people are incapable of being two or more things at the same time and keeping them straight. It's a bit like the character in Shaw's play "Getting Married" who says, "If I am to be a mother, I really cannot have a man bothering me to be a wife at the same time." A normal identity is an amalgamation of many different roles and we know that a sound identity is based on a tolerance for ambiguity. Erikson says that we must be able to live with the contradictions and confusions that are part of our daily consideration of different value systems. Another viewpoint that you might find useful comes from the work of Carl Rogers, a psychologist who has had some very interesting things to say about the difficulties we get ourselves into when our values aren't as clear as they might be.

Rogers talks about something he calls the *would-should dilemma*. He says that we all encounter this from time to time and that it causes us discomfort. Here's how it works. Given a choice between doing one of two things, we often find ourselves wanting to do one of them. This is the thing we would like to do. But at the same time, we know that we really should do something else. For example, if you are invited to go partying the night before a major exam, you may feel that you would like to go, while at the same time realize that you should study and get a good night's sleep. The people who have trouble dealing with ambiguity and who don't have firmly established identities will have the most trouble deciding what to do in situations like this.

Rogers also made some interesting observations about our value systems and their relationship to our identities. Knowing who and what you are depends a large part on what your values are and what you believe in. Normally, we always act in concert with our values.

That is, it would be unusual for a person with a fully formed identity to behave in a way that went against his or her values. When teenagers haven't decided on their values, they are likely to behave one way one day and another way the next as their values shift and change.

But to get back to Rogers, he suggests that we sometimes take in another person's values without realizing that they really aren't ours at all. He calls this introjection. Think of it as injecting another person's values. The problems arise when a person makes a decision based on what seems to be their values, but they are really somebody else's. Take for example a person who has been brought up by her parents to believe that sex is dirty, unenjoyable and something that should only be tolerated for creating children. After years of this "lie back and think of England" attitude to sex, she gets married and finds that sex is really quite pleasant. However, she feels quite guilty about enjoying it. We could say that she has an identity problem and that it stems back to a faulty value system based on her introjection of her parents' values.

Developing a sound identity is not an easy task. It can take years to accomplish and it may be fine tuned repeatedly along the way. It's no wonder that teenagers who are less experienced in life have such a tough time getting theirs together.

6. *What's the Truth About Adolescent Turmoil?*

Is adolescence the time of strife and trouble that we have made it out to be or not? What are the facts? Part of the problem lies in the widespread beliefs of some terrible stereotypes, the difficulty of determining what is normal at this age and when that crosses over into abnormality and a sort of self-fulfilling prophecy that leads us to see what we believe we should see.

Let's look at the traditional view first. As long ago as Aristotle's time, the young were seen to be a problem to their elders. Aristole himself characterized them as changeful, fickle in their desires and as transitory as they are vehement. He lamented that they were often carried away by their impulses and that if they erred in any way it was always on the side of excess and exaggeration. This traditional view has obviously been around for years and it has led us to believe that the adolescent period is one of turmoil, disruption, and maladaptive behaviour. In fact, one of the first persons to counter this storm and stress view of adolescence was Margaret Mead whose studies of Samoan adolescents indicated that adolescence was a rather tranquil experience for them. Later, Anna Freud also wrote that adolescence was a period of interruption of peaceful growth and that it was difficult to decide when the normal disruptions were symptomatic of pathological problems. Similarly, Erikson calls adolescence a normative crisis and maintains that mood swings, disruptive behaviour, and social alienation stem from the normal role diffusions that accompany the identity crisis. Anna Freud goes even further in her discussions about adolescents and warns that the well-mannered, well-behaved adolescent who never shows any of these signs is probably employing excessive defenses and not developing normally.

In summary, the traditional view of the storm and stress school is that adolescence is characterized by;

- aggression
- uncontrolled sexual urges
- low ego development
- poor identity formation
- disruptive mood swings
- difficulty with parents and authorities
- depression
- behavioral symptoms that appear to be pathological
- conflict
- restlessness

Now, what is the truth? Recent studies have shown that while some of these problems do exist, only about 7 percent of all adolescents experience significant emotional problems and that on the whole, their incidence of pathological (psychotic) problems is certainly no higher than that of the general public. In fact, the truth of the matter is that:

- adolescents normally maintain their equilibrium as they grow and develop
- they learn how to control themselves and become successful, well- adjusted adults
- anxiety, mild depression, and minor problems with parents and others in authority is normal
- the difficulty in telling whether behaviour is normal or abnormal is more due to the skill (or lack of it) on the part of those doing the diagnosis than the presence of severe problems

But, you ask, "Why do we still seem to accept the storm and stress stereotype?" There are several reasons for this. First of all, its been around for a long time and seems to be ingrained in our culture. Secondly, there have been a great many studies of deviant adolescents and we have tended to generalize from these findings. Remember, it's always much more interesting to study deviant, abnormal behaviour than a group of normal people who do nothing very exciting. Thirdly, the media has emphasized the notion that adolescents are trouble and that one can expect problems if one has the misfortune to live with a teenager.

Fortunately, teenagers while exciting and frustrating at times, can also be some of the most delightful people you'll meet and the good news is that nearly all of them grow up to be fine, normal people. We did, didn't we?

7. Sexual Identification and the Issue of Homosexuality

Our thinking about sexual development has changed over the years and we are learning more and more about sexual preferences. In fact, we are living in a time of unprecedented change in terms of both our knowledge and our attitudes about the sexes. At one time, we used to think that masculinity and femininity were two separate and distinct dimensions and that you were born with either one or the other. According to this view boys were born masculine and than developed either a strong or weak orientation on this quantity. A similar pattern applied to girls and femininity. However Sandra Bem and others have led us to realize that masculinity and femininity are not two different dimensions, but the opposite ends of a single dimension. We have also created a new term "androgeny" to describe mid-points on this scale where a person may show equal characteristics of masculinity and femininity. In the meantime, society has changed and both sexes are being encouraged to be more androgenous. Hence women are exhorted to be more masculine and to be more assertive and self-reliant while men are urged to be more nurturing and caring.

In addition, our knowledge about homosexuality has undergone some significant changes as new developments and theories have come to light. This whole issue has a strange and complex history. Homosexuality has been around since the beginning of recorded history and undoubtedly before that. The ancient Greek and Roman world accepted homosexuality as normal and it wasn't until later that it was looked upon as abnormal and abhorrent. Up to recently, we believed that homosexuals chose to be this way and that if we could only hit upon the right treatment, they could be returned to a "normal" sexual orientation. In the past, there have been some dreadful attempts to "cure" homosexuality. In the 1940s transorbital lobotomies were attempted. In this procedure, a long sharp instrument was inserted through the eye socket and moved to destroy the prefrontal lobe in the brain. This accomplished nothing. Nor did electric shock, nor aversive therapy, nor castration. Similarly psychiatry was unsuccessful and we began to realize that homosexuality was not a preference, nor was it a form of pathology. Indeed, the major psychological reference for diagnosing disorders, the Diagnostic and Statistical Manual (DSM) dropped homosexuality from its list of disorders.

More recently, biological investigations have led us to a better understanding of the biological role in homosexuality. We have learned, for example, that if newborn male rats are deprived of testosterone, they will experience female-like ovulation, while female rats deprived of testosterone will continue to develop as females. It seems that at least in rats, testosterone is as necessary for the development of a masculine brain as it is for the development of male genital organs.

Studies of the human brain have turned up evidence that suggest that there is a biological, anatomical difference between homosexuals and heterosexuals. Furthermore, it seems that there may be a prenatal link to hormone development that has an effect on sexual orientation. These kinds of studies are just beginning and the results are not conclusive at this time, nevertheless, it is clear that there is evidence that biological factors play an important role in determining sexual orientation.

If this proves to be the case, it could become a critical factor in changing our attitudes towards homosexuals and in helping them to be more readily accepted by their relatives and society in general. Our attitudes are changing now even without this evidence and if nothing else, we are talking more openly about sexual orientation. Our laws are already changing and people cannot be discriminated against on the basis of sexual preference. The mass media either reflects what's happening in society, or society reflects what it sees in the media, but in either case, it is significant that Lynn Johnson, creator of the comic strip For Better Or Worse, introduced an adolescent who has confronted his homosexuality in her strip. The comic strip is syndicated and appears in hundreds of newspapers in Canada and the USA. It's interesting to note that only a small handful of newspapers dropped the strip or ran something else.

I am not young enough to know everything.

—James M. Barrie

8. Understanding the Parental-Adolescent Conflict

By now, you should have come to the conclusion that adolescence isn't quite as bad as it's made out to be but there are periods of conflict. Most of these involve problems getting along with parents. I can't promise to help you eliminate these, but I can help you achieve a better understanding about why they happen. The basis for this improved understanding lies in knowing what to expect from adolescents and recognizing what concerns most parents have about their adolescents.

The typical teenager behaves in a surprisingly consistent way once you know what to look for. Here are some of the things you can expect.

Typical Teenage Behaviours

1. Exclusion of parents
2. New sexual feelings
3. Idealism
4. Money for me
5. Less communication
6. New loyalties and friends
7. Reduced family involvement
8. Demand for privacy
9. Exaggerated physical concerns
10. Rich fantasy life
11. Focus on the present
12. Improved grooming

- Exclusion of parents—The peer group is more important now than parents and the teenager is simply trying to achieve independence while caught in a dependency relationship with parents.

- New sexual feelings—This is when first love affairs begin and male and female bonding accelerates.

- Idealism in everything—This applies to the world in general and is accompanied by an attitude that the older generation has screwed things up. Coupled with the pseudo sophistication we mentioned earlier, this leads adolescents to believe that they could do a better job of running the zoo, school, family, your life, or anything else to which they put their mind.

- Money is used for self gratification—Living with a peer group where status is dependent upon having the latest, best, smartest, most fashionable things means that the adolescent naturally wants to buy entrance to this club. Perhaps this is where the attitude that, "he who dies with the most toys, wins" started. In any event, money and debt seem to be mutually exclusive concepts.

- Reduced communication with parents—Reduced may be too gentle here. Sometimes it's non-existent. Again, this is natural as adolescents strive for independence and autonomy. (Is there an echo of Erikson here?) In addition, they have undoubtedly learned that the less disclosed to parents, the less there is to be questioned about. Remember, this is a time of experimentation and that dreadful creature your beloved child brings home, may not really be a lifelong love and your future in-law, but simply an interesting thing your teenager is trying out.

- Shifting loyalties and new friends—As time goes on, adolescents mature as do their values, tastes, ideas, and choice of friends. Old friends drop away and are replaced by new ones who share similar interests. Remember Erikson's comments about fidelity? This is where it hits home and older adolescents adjust to the fact that their best childhood friends just don't seem to be as interesting anymore.

- Dropping out of the family—Teenagers tend to resist the family, family gatherings, contacts with relatives, and anything that takes them from their friends. Families won't return to a position of importance for some years.

- Increased demands for privacy and time alone—Strangely enough, the socially oriented adolescents want time to themselves. Usually this means distancing themselves from the family, but it can include other adolescents. Sometimes, it seems that the world is just too complex and confusing and the best recourse is to step aside for a while. Don't we all have the same desires at times?

- Exaggerated physical concerns—This is the time when one's body is changing and the teenager feels compelled to scrutinize it for abnormalities and blemishes. Adolescents worry about, are they growing fast enough, or too fast, whether their noses, ears, legs, breasts or any other parts are the right size, the right shape or attached at the right places.

- A rich fantasy life—One of the best ways to learn how to deal with desires, hopes, dreams, and fears is by fantasizing about them. It's much safer to daydream about going on a big date with a desirable person than to risk rejection and actually go out with them. This is normal and healthy.

- A focus on the here and now—Tomorrow seems like a long way off for most adolescents. They tend to live each day to the fullest and any parental discussions about, "What will happen next year and shouldn't you be making some plans for it?" are bound to be unsatisfactory.

- A change from slob to suave—It gladdens parent's hearts but leaves them puzzled when the teenage slob they have been living with, that person who never picks up after themself and thinks nothing of going out in torn jeans and dirty shirts suddenly becomes interested in personal grooming and neat clothing. Of course the maturing peer group and the opposite sex have something to do with this, and it may not turn out to be the long awaited blessing parents think as they now wait for entrance to the bathroom or shower.

Now what about the parental side of the equation? Just as parents don't understand adolescents, it works the other way too. It would be helpful if the adolescents knew that just having a teenager raises a number of surprisingly common concerns in the minds of their parents. The first of these is simple fear. A fear that their child is entering a world that is more complex, more dangerous, and less understandable than the one they inhabited at their age. Today's parents certainly didn't have to face the same kind of drug concerns, AIDS, and the bewildering choice of career alternatives that their children encounter. We tend to fear what we don't understand and it's natural for parents to be concerned and to feel that their children don't have enough experience, insight, or appreciation for the issues that are facing them. I think our parents must have felt that way too.

Secondly, the fact that their adolescents are moving away from them and seeking more independence leaves parents with a feeling of a loss of control. They are concerned that they will be unable to protect their offspring from dangers and that they will not know in advance what they are getting into so they can warn and prepare them for what lies ahead.

Thirdly, parents want to help their children avoid doing what they did at their age, making the same kinds of mistakes, missing opportunities, making the wrong choices, taking the same dumb chances we did.

Fourthly, parents feel a sense of loss. Often this is the loss of the little boy or girl that was such a delight, or a loss of innocence, and sometimes it manifests itself in a sense of a loss of time remaining as the parent must now confront the fact that their child is becoming an adult. It's hard to continue to think of oneself as a young parent when your son wears all your clothing, knows more about something than you do, and is bigger and taller than you are. Where does the time go?

Finally, there is a sense of helplessness as the parents come to terms with the realization that whatever kind of job they have done raising this adolescent, there is nothing much more they can do.

Nevertheless, as parents and most adolescents come to understand, the parent-child roles are very strong and hard to break. Most parents act like parents all their lives and feel entitled or obligated to comment on most aspects of their child's life, seemingly forever. I think this just goes with the territory. However, there is more truth than poetry in the sign I have in my office at the university. It reads, "The next best thing to a good education is a pushy mother."

9. Where to Find More Information

Baldwin, B. A. "Puberty and Parents: Understanding your early adolescent." *PACE Magazine.* Oct., 1986. p. 13+

Bem, S. L. *Beyond Androgyny: Some Presumptuous Prescriptions for a Liberated Sexual Identity.* (Keynote address for APA/NUIMH conference on the Research Needs of Women.) Madison, Wisconsin, May 31, 1975.

Burr, C." Homosexuality and Biology." *The Atlantic Monthly.* Mar, 1993, 271, 3. p. 47–65.

Flaste, R. "The Myth about Teen-Agers." *New York Times Magazine.* Oct. 9, 1988. p. 19+.

Goldberg, H. *The New Male-Female Relationship.* New York: Morrow. 1983.

Oldham, D. G. "Adolescent Turmoil: a Myth revisited." *Journal of Continuing Education in Psychiatry,* 1978, *39,* 3. p. 23–32.

Rogers, C. R. *On Becoming a Person.* Boston: Houghton Mifflin. 1961.

chapter 4

The Young Adulthood Period

The value of marriage is not that adults produce children but that children produce adults.

—Peter De Vries

---

1. The Developmental Tasks

This can be a long period with a great many things happening in it, and there are many normal developmental tasks that the young adult has to be able to accomplish. We're going to start with the normal tasks as identified by Havighurst. You'll note that since these were created in the 1970s, they focus on the traditional nuclear family. Here are some of the major ones:

- Selecting and courting a mate—Today this means finding someone who will be a lifelong friend, advisor, lover, and business partner.

- Learning to live with someone—Of course having found a mate, one must learn to live with them. This isn't as easy at it sounds and the first year of marriage is usually one that requires great adjustment on the part of both people.

- Starting a family—This will make a significant change in the relationship and indeed the birth of the first child is the single most disruptive event that will occur. Life will never be quite the same again as roles change, new needs appear, additional responsibilities are created, etc.
- Rearing children—This involves meeting a host of demands that most people never clearly anticipate.
- Learning to manage a home—This includes selecting a home, furnishing and paying for it too. But it also includes all those other things such as cooking, cleaning, shopping, home maintenance, and paying the bills.
- Getting started in a career—This is an undertaking that could take up most of a person's time in itself. What's more, the choice of an occupation can be critical to the future happiness of the individuals and as a couple.

  Finding a congenial social group—Since we are social animals, we like to congregate with others. One of the tasks now is to find a social circle of people with whose interests we share and that we like.
- Taking on some sort of civic responsibility—Usually, we get drawn into the organizations we are part of. For example, most parents take a greater interest in the school system once they have children in it.

But what about the young adult who is not married? Aren't there developmental tasks that apply to them too? Of course there are and the following list applies to all young adults regardless of their marital status.

- Developing competence—This refers to the application of skills, acquiring of new skills and polishing and refining skills.
- Achieving autonomy—This is not mere independence, it means being able to fend for oneself, to be able to be self-

reliant. I see this in action every fall when the first year students leave home for the first time and come to the university. Eventually, around mid- October, the supply of clean clothes runs out and it's time to wash everything. Often this is literally what happens and everything is tossed in together with the result that the students appear in pink jeans and shirts for a while until they get it figured out.

- Developing and implementing values—The value system is dynamic, not static, and subject to changes and fine tuning as one ages.

- Forming an identity—You didn't really think this was finished in adolescence did you? The young adult takes on many new roles as a result of marriage, getting a job, having a child, etc., and each of them involve learning new behaviours.

- Integrating sexuality into life—This may involve getting married, but even if it does, the young adult must decide with whom, when, and under what circumstances to have sex.

- Learning to use leisure time—At first glance this may seem like a silly thing to have to learn, but the young adult probably has more free time now and the money to do something with it than ever before. This is where decisions must be made about whether to travel, go to a cottage, start snowmobiling, skiing, take up bicycling, etc.

2. The Life Cycle of the Family

Just as we have a life cycle theory for the lifespan, Sonya Rhodes has developed an interesting and useful theory concerning the life cycle of a family. To be sure, she must have been thinking about the traditional, nuclear family when she developed her ideas, but the concepts are still valid and help us understand what is likely to happen in a family setting. Like Erikson, she says that each stage is characterized by an expectable crisis that can be resolved for the better or for the worse. But before we get to the theory itself, let me draw your attention to some rather basic characteristics of most families.

1. The family is a symbiotic relationship in that everybody in it both takes something from and contributes something to the family unit. The members of a family are normally interdependent and rely on each other for certain things. Hence a change for one family member will change things for everyone.

2. The family strives to maintain itself and to set boundaries to accomplish this. That is, it protects itself and its members, pulls together and closes ranks when under attack.

3. The family is a flexible, adaptive and equilibrium seeking unit. It can and does change as time goes on and it will adapt to change, but its members try to achieve a sense of balance and equilibrium in the process.

4. The family is a task oriented unit and performs tasks that satisfy its own needs and that of the society and culture in which it exists. In this way it serves to socialize its members.

Now, what about the seven stages that Rhodes proposed? While this too is a stage theory, there are no specific ages for any of them

Rhode's Life Cycle of the Family

Stage	Period	Expected Crisis
1	Before children	Intimacy vs. idealization or disillusionment
2	The childbearing years	Replenishment vs. turning inward
3	After childbearing and preschool ages	Individuation of family members vs. pseudomutual organization
4	Families with teenagers	Companionship vs. isolation
5	Children are leaving home	Regrouping vs. binding or expulsion
6	First post-parental period	Rediscovery vs. despair
7	Second post-parental preiod	Mutual aid vs. uselessness

except in the most general way. You'll soon realize that the theory works best for the traditional family and that it is harder to apply it to families that spread their child rearing over many years or blended or reconstituted families formed when there is a remarriage of one or both partners. Nevertheless, Rhode's ideas still give us some useful insights into what is happening in most families.

1. *Intimacy versus Idealization or Disillusionment*—This stage applies to the first period in a marriage when the couple have come together. The major task to be achieved is that of becoming intimate with each other. The success of this is dependent upon having a realistic perception of the other partner as opposed to having an idealized, unrealistic view about the other person. If someone enters a marriage with dreams of never ending romantic love, hot passion, and a fairy tale existence, one is in for a rude awakening.

Since the first year of marriage is normally a period of great upheaval, adjustment and conflict, entering into it with unrealistic ideals can only lead to trouble. If the couple fail to achieve intimacy, they may suffer disillusionment and disappointment. Let's take a simple example concerning the kinds of adjustments one has to make in this first year. I'm an only child and everyone in my house woke up easily and quickly in the morning. Naturally, I assumed that everyone in the world was like this so it was a great surprise when I discovered that my wife didn't leap out of bed, ready to face the day just as I did. Similarly, she found it difficult to understand why I liked to have a short nap anytime I felt so inclined, since no one in her experience except her aging grandfather ever slept in the middle of the day.

Couples always enter a marriage with a certain amount of idealization and most move to a true Eriksonian type of intimacy. However, there are at least three ways in which they can tackle this issue. First, one of the members can refuse to adjust or demand that the other person accommodate to their wishes. If they do not or can not, one person can withdraw and the marriage fails. Secondly, the couple can agree that they simply won't address or acknowledge the problem. While this can work for short siestas, it won't work for more serious problems such as who handles the money. This approach generally results in rigidity, unhappiness, and continuing conflict. The third approach is that of discussing the problem and coming up with a mutually satisfying solution.

2. *Replenishment versus Turning Inward*—This stage applies to the childbearing years. It begins with the birth of the first child and ends when the last child enters school. The major task here is how to supply the children with all of the nurturance and attention they need while not draining the main caregivers. That is, the children certainly must be attended to but who cares for the caretakers? Continually giving of oneself without a chance to refuel, recharge one's batteries, or simply have time for one's own needs can really drain a person. The danger is that either the most responsible caregiver (usually the mother) will become exhausted or that the increased attention to the children will leave the father feeling abandoned. In either case, one or both of the parents may turn inward and away from the family to satisfy their own needs.

3. *Individuation of Family Members versus Pseudomutual Organization*—Don't be confused or put off by the terms. They really make great sense when you understand what they mean and if nothing else they sound very impressive at cocktail parties. This stage applies to families with children who are past the preschool years but whose children are not yet teenagers. These families must turn their attention from family concerns to the concerns of the family members who are becoming more independent and autonomous. A child's identity is not defined solely by being a member of a family. They have a growing number of other interests and are becoming less dependent on the family for everything. This period can become a problem for mothers who find that they are no longer needed as much

by their children and who have no other role to satisfy a need to be needed.

The idea of pseudomutual organization is that of a family that strives to preserve cohesion and harmony while denying the growing independence of the children or the parents. This happens when a family mistakes closeness for cohesion. This can happen when the family (usually the parents) have decided that certain standards and behaviours will always be followed by the family. For example, they may feel that it is essential that the family associate only with members of their own race, culture, or religion. Problems immediately surface when a family member is discovered to be friends with someone who doesn't fit the criteria. The danger is that the offending family members (often the children) will seem to go along with the family dogma in order to keep peace, but in reality follow their own consciences. Hence, it only seems that the family values are being preserved.

4. *Companionship versus Isolation*—This stage applies to families with adolescent children and the task to handle here is the ability of all family members, but especially the teenagers, to develop companionship outside and inside the family. The teenager side of the equation is easy to see, but this stage also applies to the parents, who now have time to rediscover each other and to renew their marriage. If this isn't possible and comfortable companionship isn't achieved, it can and will lead to a sense of isolation.

5. *Regrouping versus Binding or Expulsion*—This stage applies to families whose children are leaving home. The major crisis here is that of adjusting to the independence of the children, their move outside the family home, and coping with this natural need for separation. The task is to allow the children to leave without attaching apron strings, or unreasonable restraints with the parents and the siblings who are still at home. If this is done successfully, the family regroups as a new mix of those who are

still left and the children who have become adults and who now live outside of the family home. It causes a problem when the parents try to bind or maintain control over those who are leaving and insist on adherence to the old parental standards. Sometimes when the children resist efforts to restrain them, the parents withdraw their support and expel the children from the family. This is a sort of, "my way or hit the highway" attitude on the part of the parents and it never works.

6. *Rediscovery versus Despair*—The last two stages in Rhodes theory cover the two phases when the family unit has changed in that there are no children at home. It's interesting to note that these two periods cover approximately 50% of the time that couple are together. In any event, this stage begins when the last child has moved out and the tasks now are for the marriage partners to rediscover each other and deal with the fact that they will be living without the children and with only each other for some years to come. A satisfactory resolution of this period is a revival of the marriage and a mutual attempt by both the parents and the children to maintain relationships. If this doesn't occur, there is a danger that there will be a feeling known as the empty nest. A related task to be attended to is that of forging a new relationship with one's children based on an adult to adult interaction rather than the old adult to child pattern. Obviously, rediscovery is good and a failure to achieve this can lead to despair.

7. *Mutual Aid versus Uselessness*—This is the final stage of the original family and covers the period from the parents' retirement until their deaths. The major task here is to establish a mutual aid system in which both the parents and their children rely on each other as the need arises. Parents normally need to feel that they are still able to assist their children and that they have an important role to play as grandparents. But as time goes on, the roles will slowly reverse and the parents will become more dependent on their children. It's probably accurate to say that the parents are more subject to a feeling of

uselessness than their children if things don't work out, but feelings of resentment on either side are common where the mutual aid system falters.

Love is the word used to label the sexual excitement of the young, the habituation of the middle-aged, and the mutual dependence of the old.

—John Ciardi

---

3. Marriage, Satisfaction and Potential Conflicts

George Bernard Shaw made a very interesting point when he observed that just when two people are under the influence of the most violent, most insane, most delusive, and most transient of passions they go through a marriage ceremony in which they swear that they will remain in that excited, abnormal, and exhausting condition until death do them part. Most people enter a marriage this way and we probably wouldn't want it any other way. However, it does set up a series of elevated expectations for us and we are disappointed to find that this fever pitch doesn't last forever. If we look at a special set of developmental tasks pertinent to married couples, we can see that there are many things that they must learn how to do if they are to survive very long with much harmony. These tasks include such things as:

- Achieving intimacy—this includes adjusting to the other person's personal habits and temperamental differences as well as learning how to fulfill the sexual and emotional needs of one another.

- Determining how to make decisions—there is a certain amount of jockeying for position and power in the early days of most marriages as the couple decide who is going to be responsible for making what kinds of decisions. The questions of who will take responsibility for the cooking, cleaning, shopping, lawn, and home maintenance are fairly easy and have traditionally been decided along pretty stereotypic lines. However, this is changing and when it comes to the question of who does the banking, tax preparation, investing and spending the money for things like cars and holidays, the couple may have to quickly learn how to cooperate, negotiate and compromise.

- Working out extra family relationships—This refers to getting along with the parents, in-laws and assorted other relatives. This can be a very difficult problem and many newly married couples find themselves racing from one parental home to the other at Christmas, Mother's Day, and Easter as they try to satisfy everyone with their presence. We knocked ourselves out the first two Christmases we were married even though we desperately wanted to have our own celebration at our apartment, but we didn't know how to extricate ourselves from our parents' expectations. We managed to break the cycle by going to Nassau the third year.

- Accomplishing companionship—This is nothing more than the task of learning to live and think as "we" rather an "I." It's one thing to see your intended for a few hours every few days, but it's quite another to actually live with them 24 hours a day. Consequently, couples must learn to work, play, plan, talk, eat and sleep together. This necessitates sharing space, time, interests, belongings, and ideas, as well as the bathroom.

- Settling on a social life—This includes decisions about whose friends will you socialize with, learning to entertain as a couple, planning and executing joint activities, and what kinds of social activities you will participate in as a couple.

- Learning how to fight—Let's be honest, no couple exists 365 days a year without getting annoyed at each other. But do they know how to settle their differences? Some couples allow one person to control most things in the marriage, others continually struggle for dominance while some learn how to get the issues out into the open and then reach a mutually agreeable settlement. The first two methods invariably lead to anger and resentment, but not everyone knows how to approach conflicts effectively.

The strength of a nation is derived from the integrity of its homes.

—Confucius (c. 551–479 B.C.)

---

4. The Importance of the Family and Why We Have Reached A Turning Point

For years we have thought that while the traditional family was important, it was not good for anyone to have a marriage in trouble continue and that if it did end in divorce, the effects on everyone, including the children would be short lived and minor. However, more and more studies are now showing that the breakup of the traditional two-parent family is very harmful, especially for children and that these effects last for many years. As we learn more about this and more evidence is amassed, it is quite likely that we will see a return to older values concerning marriage and that divorce and having children out-of-wedlock will be frowned upon and discouraged. In fact, it can be convincingly argued that society cannot afford to allow the family to disintegrate at the present rate.

Consider these facts. Before World War II more than 80% of all children grew up in traditional, two-parent homes. But by 1980 only

50% would spend their entire childhood in an intact family. The effects of this are quite alarming for everyone when you realize that compared with a two-parent home, children from single parent homes are six times as likely to be poor, three times as likely to have emotional and behavioural problems, and more likely to drop out of school, get pregnant while teenagers and find themselves in trouble with the law. In addition, recent research has shown that children do not recover quickly after a marital breakup and that the effects may last well into adulthood.

In previous generations, marital disruptions were held in check by a society that did not sanction divorce, separation, or out-of-wedlock births. In fact, anyone who became involved in any of these things was stigmatized by our society and social institutions. My parents, for example, did not know a single couple who were divorced, nor did my wife's parents. Before the invention of the birth control pill, the fear of an unwanted pregnancy was one of the things that kept most young people on the straight and narrow. If a girl did get pregnant, it went without saying that the boy would marry her, and shotgun weddings were shameful, but not uncommon.

In the 60s, attitudes changed in our society and divorces became easier to obtain and less shameful. Where the divorce rate had been steady at about 10 per 1000 marriages, it suddenly rose to more than double that and by 1974, divorce passed death as the number one cause of marital dissolution. The same thing happened to out-of-wedlock births and they increased 500% between 1960 and 1990. At the present time, half of all marriages end in divorce and even those who cohabit and then marry or those who remarry are even more likely to have their marriages end in divorce.

The result of all this is that more and more children are being raised in single parent families or in step-parent families, or a series of them. At the present time, fewer than half the children born now will live in an intact family for their entire childhood and one out of every four will become part of a step-parent family. As these trends developed, our attitudes about what was best for both the parents and the children also shifted. Where we once thought that the breakup of the family was bad for children, we now said that this was in everybody's best interest and that the effects were short lived anyhow. As a result, there was a shift in focus from what's best for the child, to what's best for the adults. This is still the case today, but I suspect it won't stay that way much longer. We are still being fed the old message from Hollywood and the media who delight in telling us how celebrities have shucked off their marriages, shacked up with someone new or are busy discovering themselves while their children are handling it all very well and in a most mature fashion. What nonsense! The epitome of this kind of thing are sit-coms that promote single parenthood, out-of-wedlock children and a sort of no-fault parenthood where the focus is on the joys of creating children and no one thinks about how they will be raised. In fact, there are many cases where the intact, traditional, two-parent family is portrayed as something sinister and pathological where incest, abuse, and alcoholism run rampant.

The danger here is that people mistake this news as a diatribe against single parents and people who want out of damaging, abusive marriages. This would be like shooting the messenger because you don't like the message. No one is suggesting that people should stay married at all costs. In fact, research has shown that 80% of divorced women and 50% of divorced men say they are much better off not being married, or at least not being married to their former partner. The point is that we seem to have shifted our attention away from what's best for children to what's good for the adults. While in fact, those things that contribute to the adult's happiness may be in direct opposition to the child's happiness now and in the future. It's quite natural for divorced parents to enjoy their newfound freedom and independence and to search for new outlets, develop new interests, and look for new partners. Consequently, they tend to invest more time and effort looking after their own needs while the needs of their children take a back seat.

This was brought home to me very directly in a film about childhood that I use with my classes. One of the scenes shows a young man; he looks to be in his late teens, talking about his divorced mother and how he has taken over the raising of the family. As he said it, "One minute I'm telling my little sister to eat her supper, get her clothes ready for school the next day, and helping her with her homework. The next minute, I'm asking my Mom about the guy she's seeing now. "Who is he? Does she like him? Will he be staying the night?" "But", he says, "I have no one to go to when I have a problem or just need to talk." He also makes the point that you see a lot of sex in a broken home, but not much love. Not much of a model for a future parent, is it.

So, what is the truth about disintegrating families and the effect on children? There are a number of places that are studying this issue now and some of their findings are highly disturbing. Results from the California Children of Divorce Study indicate that children simply do not "get over" the divorce of their parents and that the effects last and last. The study found that more than a third of the children of divorce were moderately or severely depressed five years after the divorce and that ten years later a significant number of the children who were now in their teens were troubled, disturbed, and drifting. The researchers also found effects that lasted fifteen years after the break-up.

But even if the children manage to cope fairly well, there are other insidious effects that we are just recognizing now. The parent-child relationship is permanently altered. This applies to both the mothers and the fathers, but the father-child relationship is often damaged the most severely. In an intact family, a child moves from one parent to the other learning from each and developing skills and attitudes that are necessary for normal development. But all too often the children seldom see one of the parents after a divorce; there is decreasing communication and diminishing psychological and financial support. This applies to both parents, but even more so to fathers. Even where the children live with the mother, research has shown that the mother-child bond is weakened. As a result, children in disrupted families are twice as likely to drop out of school, to underachieve while attending school and to be behaviour problems in the school. In fact, the case can and is being made that one of the major reasons for under achievement in our schools is due to the increasing number of children from broken homes. School officials report so many of these children are so caught up with what is happening in their families and so emotionally distraught that they are incapable of doing normal school work.

As if this wasn't bad enough, the studies also present damming evidence that most of the increases in child poverty and an overwhelming majority of juvenile crime can be attributed to disintegrating families. The rise in crime, especially juvenile and violent juvenile crime is absolutely frightening. It has been reported that more than 70% of all juveniles in American state reform institutions come from fatherless homes. Unfortunately, single mother homes are only slightly better. The effects are so strong that even when one controls for income and race, family configuration comes out as the primary factor in juvenile crime.

Well, having presented all of this disturbing information, where does that leave us? On the brink of a major attitude shift I think. To be sure the facts aren't all in, but there is certainly an overwhelming body of respectable research all pointing in the same direction and I am confident that you will be seeing more and more attention being paid to this issue in the popular press. Watch for it on your local newsstand. In addition, I think we are about to see a significant change in attitudes about the importance of the family. Things can change fairly quickly once people become aware and educated about an issue. Look for example how our attitudes and laws have changed about smoking. In the meantime, if you are married, you may want to think about your obligation to your children. If you are about to get married, you'd better discuss the importance of staying together and if you are already divorced, you might want to think about how you can best protect yourself and your children from some of these effects. We seem to be rather thin on suggestions for what to do after the fact, but that too will change as we realize what we are up against. In the meantime, you might take the lead from one of my married students who went home after our class on this topic and told her husband "If you ever mention the word divorce in this house, you're toast!"

> *No man knows his true character until he has run out of gas, purchased something on the installment plan and raised an adolescent.*
>
> —Mercelene Cox

5. Some of the Myths About Being a Parent

While we are bursting bubbles, let me give you some interesting information about some of the myths that have sprung up about being a parent. Many people unconsciously believe these things are true, but they are not. Knowing the facts can help you avoid a few problems and a lot of guilt.

Parenting Myths

1. Babies save marriages
2. Your children will be like you
3. Your children will care for you
4. Parents will be respected
5. Parents can live through their children
6. Parents can mold their children
7. It's the parents' fault when a child fails
8. Mothers are better than fathers
9. Parenting is instinctual

1. Having a baby will save a failing marriage. Well after reading the section above I probably don't need to add anything more here, but like all academics I will anyway. Marriage can be very demanding at the best of times and the birth of a child is always a disruptive influence in any marriage. If a couple is already having problems, adding a baby to the situation certainly won't improve it. In fact, it's almost guaranteed to make it worse.

2. Your children will be like you, look like you, and think and act like you. Well, they may look like you, or a relative somewhere in your genetic past and they may even share some of your traits and personality characteristics. But they will grow up as individuals, doing things you never dreamed of and living in a world that we can scarcely imagine.

3. Your children will take care of you in your old age. This used to be the case, but unless you instill your children with hefty doses of ideas about honor and obligation, you can't be sure that they will take care of you. Not only have our social welfare systems encouraged us to leave that responsibility up to others, it may be impossible for your children to take care of you in the style to which you have become accustomed. Indeed, it has been suggested that the current young generation will not be able to live as well as their parents.

4. Parents will get respect and obedience from their children. While we probably all assume that our children will be this way, it doesn't always turn out like this. It's not likely to happen during adolescence, but the respect part at least often returns later.

5. Having a child gives parents a second chance to achieve what they failed to achieve. Certainly not. How many lives have been made miserable by parents who have pushed their children into activities that only they were interested in, or towards professions that they wish they had taken up.

6. Parents can mold their children if they apply the right techniques. Perhaps, but only to a point and it never turns out the

way you think it should. Besides, it assumes that the parents really do know what's best for their children at all times. We used to believe this when the TV program "Father Knows Best" was popular, but who accepts that now?

7. It is the parents' fault when a child fails. Not necessarily. Parents can only do their best for their children. They can't lead their lives for them and even if they did, who among us feels that we are so great at living that we never made any mistakes. Remember, we learn just as much and often more from failures as we do from our successes.

8. Mothers are better parents that fathers. Sometimes it seems that way, but the truth of the matter is that there are just as many good and bad examples on both sides. No one sex has an advantage here. After all, it's a learned behaviour and anybody can learn how to do it better.

9. Parenting is instinctual and requires no training. Unfortunately this just isn't the case. There is reason to doubt whether there is even such a thing as a maternal instinct and when it comes to parenting skills, no one is born with them. Like most other behaviours, this is something that we learn, usually from seeing others model the behaviours, but the fact that we have parenting courses and books such as Dr. Spock's baby book is testament to the fact that it doesn't come naturally.

The great secret of successful marriage is to treat all disasters as incidents and none of the incidents as disasters.

—Harold Nicholson

---

6. *Where to Go for More Information*

Baldwin, B. A. "Positive Parenting: How to Avoid Raising Cornucopia Kids." *PACE Magazine,* Nov., 1988. p. 16+.

Dyer, E. D. "Parenthood as Crisis: a Re-study." *Marriage and Family Living.* 1963, *25.* p. 196–201.

Gibson, N. *Separation and Divorce: a Woman's Survival Guide.* Alberta: Hurtig Publishers. 1986.

Kitson, G. C., K. B. Babri and M. J. Roach. "Who Divorces and Why: a Review." *Journal of Family Issues.* Sep., 1985, *6, 3.*

Kressel, K. "Patterns of Coping in Divorce." *Family Relations.* 1980, *9.* p. 234–40.

McCubbin, H.I. and R. F. Figley. (eds.) *Stress and the Family: Volume 1 Coping with Normative Transitions.* New York: Brunner/Mazel Inc. 1983.

Rhodes, S. L. "A Developmental Approach to the Life Cycle of the Family." *Family Service Association of America,* from *Social Caseworks* May 1977, *58,* 5. p. 301–311.

Singer, L. S. *The Crisis That Shapes Your Marriage.* New York: Grosset and Dunlop. 1980.

Skinner, D. A. "Dual-Career Family Stress and Coping." *Family Relations* 1980, 29. p. 473–481.

Wallerstein, J. S. "Children after Divorce: Wounds that don't Heal." *The New York Times Magazine,* Jan. 22, 1989, p. 19–21.

Whitehead, B. D. "Dan Quayle Was Right." *The Atlantic Monthly.* Apr., 1993, *271,* 4. p. 47–84.

chapter 5

What's Happening to Adults at Mid-Life?

The first half of our life is ruined by our parents and the second half by our children.

—Clarence Darrow

1. The Developmental Tasks

This list of developmental tasks is a little shorter at this age and of course the time to complete it is a little longer. In a way, this is typical of what happens in middle-age. You have more time to make some of the adjustments. Some of the things that normally developing adults must face are:

1. Achieving civic and social responsibility—This refers to the continuation of the process that began in young adulthood but which now takes on a larger measure of importance as adults move into more responsible positions in their communities and community organizations. It also happens because by now, these adults and their opinions are more respected and they are more skilled at handling people.

2. Establishing and maintaining economic stability—This is normally the period of peak earning power for adults, especially if they are part of a dual income family. It is also the time when

the economic demands of the family are diminishing. All the major purchases have been made at this stage and the adults are in a period of replacement of things (like cars and roofs) rather than first time buyers.

3. Assisting older children—There may still be the odd teenager at home at the beginning of this period, but they will likely be moving out and establishing their own homes. Even when (and if) the children leave home, the parents find themselves involved in new kinds of relationships with their adult offspring.

4. Enhancing or redeveloping intimacy with one's spouse. It has been said rather tongue in cheek that life truly begins for the middle-aged couple when the dog dies and the children leave home. This is the time when the couple realize that they have some delightful years ahead of them and that they can devote more time to each other.

5. Adjusting to aging—Now is the time when the physical and psychological effects of aging really become apparent. Men's hair is a little thinner, there are a few more wrinkles and it's a little harder to bounce back after strenuous activity. My doctor says he gets a flood of calls every spring from adults who he says are suffering from what he calls A.A.—Aging Athlete.

6. Accepting and adjusting to one's aging parents—We always seem to assume that our parents will be there for us and that they will go on forever, but at this age, we realize that they are getting older and may be more dependent upon us than they were before.

7. Developing leisure time activities—Adults at this period have more disposable income and are interested in ways to use it for the maximum enjoyment. For some, that winter break in the sunny south becomes very appealing.

8. Developing deep and mutually supportive friendships—Usually at this time, adults have developed a stable group of friends the same age. This social group takes on new importance.

9. Preparing for retirement—Perhaps "preparing" is too optimistic a term here, but as one ages it's natural that thoughts turn to retirement and dreams of what it will be like. This accelerates as one's associates retire.

2. *Whose Theories are Useful for This Age?*

Here again, I'm not going to give you an exhaustive run down of the major theorists because you can find everything you need in the references I've listed. Besides, as you'll quickly realize, we simply don't have any comprehensive theories that explain everything that is happening at this age. However, I want to direct your attention to the work of Levinson Vaillant, Gould, and Neugarten.

Levinson developed a very interesting theory concerning the development of adult men. But note that he has never claimed to say anything about women. Levinson is best known for his book *The Seasons of a Man's Life* and his popularization of the notion of a mid-life crisis. He says that around the age of 40, men appraise where they are in life and what they've done, confront their own mortality, take some corrective actions and deal with four major concerns. These concerns Levinson presents are polarities that a man must wrestle with. In the Young-Old polarity, a man must consider how he feels about his age and come to terms with the idea that he has now lived longer than he has left to live. The Destruction-Creation polarity involves the realization that we all have the power to act destructively towards people, including our loved ones, but that we are also capable of being constructive and we can contribute to our world. The third polarity of Masculine-Feminine reflects the realization that men have a mixture of both elements and it may be appropriate now to ease up on one and allow the other to show. The fourth polarity is that of Attachment-Separateness and involves a consideration of how important others may be to the man and how important it may be to have privacy and be responsible only to oneself.

Roger Gould also has some interesting things to say about adult development and unlike Levinson, his theory applies to both men and women. He identified seven stages and linked them to broad-age categories and suggested the major development tasks as follows:

Stage 1 16–18—wanting to leave parental control

Stage 2 18–22—leaving the family, a peer group orientation

Stage 3 22–28—developing independence, committing to career and a family and children

Stage 4 29–34—questioning the self, role confusion, potential marital dissatisfaction

Stage 5 35–43—an urgency to complete life goals, awareness of the limitations of time, realignment of goals

Stage 6 43–53—settling down and accepting one's life

Stage 7 53–60—more tolerance, acceptance of past, less negativism, general mellowing

You can see the similarity to Erikson and Levinson—can't you?

George Vaillant's major contribution in this area is that he suggested two additional stages for Erikson's theory. One of these, he says, should be inserted in the age 23 to 35 year period. He calls this "career consolidation" and says it is the time when a person works very hard at getting their career in order and in climbing the organizational structure they are now caught up in. His second addition is for the 45 to 55 year old period. He terms this "keeping the meaning versus rigidity." He suggests (like Levinson) that at this time, adults figure out whether their life goals have been attained and if not, how to accept life for what it is. At the same time, they try to make some sense out of their existence and work at avoiding a certain rigidity to life.

3. Is Middle-Age Something to Fear?

Just what is middle-age and what does it involve? Unfortunately, we have no clear idea of when it begins and there are certainly no rites of passage that tell us when we have reached this stage. Chronologically, the mid-point in the North American lifespan occurs at about 36, yet we typically do not consider that a person has reached middle-age until they are at least 40. Since there are no satisfactory marker events to tell us when we are middle-aged, we have developed a great many tongue-in-cheek expressions to help us pin it down. Ogden Nash said that middle-age is when you have met so many people that everyone you meet reminds you of somebody else. Somebody else put it this way, "Middle-age is when you get out of the shower and are glad the mirror is fogged."

But the truth of the matter is that people in North America live at least ten years longer than our ancestors did at the turn of the century and we are living better and are healthier now than they were at their mid-point of life. Nevertheless, people tend to become worried and anxious when they realize they are middle-aged. This seems to be because we feel older and are concerned about where we are in life and how much time we have left. In other words, it's a mental state and we can either look at it positively or negatively. One of the saddest things to see is the person who fights this natural progression every step of the way and does their darndest to retain the appearance of youth or who has a juvenile mentality. If the truth were known, most of the world's greatest achievements were accomplished by people in the middle years and beyond.

However, it is natural to become aware of death in a very personal way at this time since no one who has reached 40 hasn't experienced the death of a close relative or friend. This can be especially shocking if the death occurs to someone your own age or younger. When this happens it is quite appropriate to consider one's own mortality and to see if you have accomplished all the things you have wanted. This is a very dangerous question and it usually results in an unsatisfactory answer. As John Stuart Mill said, "Ask yourself if you are happy and you will soon cease to be so." It would be far better if we looked at mid-life as a time of opportunity, reduced pressure to compete and a chance to seek renewal and further growth and development. Middle-age is a state of mind and while many people do fear it and don't know how to handle it, it's up to us to decide what to make of it. As our population ages and we focus more attention on the adult period of life, I think we'll see more positive information about middle-age and a decrease in our negative attitudes towards it.

4. Is there Really Any Such Thing as a Mid-Life Crisis?

Much of the bad press and negative thinking about mid-life stems from the fact that we have heard so much about the mid-life crisis. This is a term that has crept into our language fairly recently, popularized by Levinson's work and the media who delight in comedies about men and women who turn 40 and then do something completely unexpected, wild, and bizarre. Movies like "10" and "Middle-age Crazy" only serve to fuel the fire. Let's take a hard look at the facts.

There may be something appealing about the idea of a fixed progression of stages of development that all adults go through. This would enable us to measure our progress against a standard and see if we are where we should be. It would also enable us to make more sense out of all the things that happen to us as adults. But the truth of the matter is that there is no such clear pattern of adult development. Bernice Neugarten and her researchers at the University of Chicago have been studying adult development for years trying to find consistent patterns. But she says that "The primary consistency we have found is a lack of consistency. We have had great trouble clustering people into age brackets that are characterized by particular conflicts; the conflicts won't stay put and neither will the people."

Part of the problem is that we are accustomed to thinking about people of a certain age as being very much alike. All one-year-old children are very much the same and we have even developed neat terms to categorize specific ages as the terrible twos, fearsome fours, friendly fives, sociable sixes, noisy nines, etc. But trying to do this for adults just doesn't work. As Neugarten points out, there is a fanning out process at work as we age and people become increasingly different as they grow older and experience a myriad of things. This supports her contention that we have become an age-irrelevant society in that where we once knew whether we were "on time" in terms of society's expectations for what we ought to be doing at any given age, this no longer applies. Hence we have 20-year-old mayors, 35- year-old grandmothers, 50-year-old mothers, 60-year-old fathers, 75-year- old students and 55-year-old retrees.

The consequence of all this is that for most of us, we no longer know or care about what we are supposed to be doing at any age and when we do stop to think about where we are in life and how we are progressing, we can decide for ourselves whether we want to be depressed about it or not. The danger is in believing that we really *ought* to have a mid-life crisis and that there is something wrong with us if we don't have one. I think there is a very good case to be made for the fact that you can only have a mid- life crisis if you have the time and money to afford one. Most of us are too busy with the normal challenges of life to go looking for more of them.

5. Can there be a Mid-Career Crisis?

The existence of a mid-life crisis is somewhat in doubt, but a related phenomenon, the mid-career crisis seems to hit many people. Consider this scenario.

Harry is in his early 40s. Married with two teenagers, he has been with his firm for 18 years. He is director of marketing, having risen from the sales ranks. He is also bored, discontent, and depressed, but he doesn't know why. When he wakes up in the morning, all he can think of is "Can I stand to do this job and work with these people for another 20 years? Is this all there is to life?"

Harry is suffering from a mid-career crisis and he is not alone. While accurate figures are hard to obtain, it is estimated that up to 40 percent of men change jobs between the ages of 40 and 60. This also applies to women who have been working for most of their adult lives. This means that vast numbers of working men and women are unhappy and unproductive in what they are doing and it is probable that these frustrations will spill over into family and non-working relationships, resulting in more discontent, rebellion, job changes, divorces, affairs, and in some cases, suicides. Mid-career crises don't happen to everyone, but they could and middle-aged people are the prime targets. Middle-aged men and women are likely to be enjoying their highest levels of income and job status, so what do they have to be unhappy about?

Psychologists studying this age group have found that the middle years are often a period of internal turmoil. It is a time of reassessment of one's life and a time for taking stock of where one is and where one hoped or expected to be by this age. Often, it is a time when one must adjust idealistic hopes to the realistic possibilities that remain.

If you had hoped to be at least a vice president, or department head or hold some other position by now and you haven't made it yet, it is normal to begin asking yourself whether you will ever get that job and to begin to wonder if perhaps you have gone as far as you can.

First of all, you have to face the fact that you are getting older. The realization that you have probably lived more years than you have left to live may be hard to accept, even depressing. If you have children, they are likely to be teenagers who are leaving home, starting careers, starting families or all of the above. It may even be the case that your children are doing very well indeed and it looks like they will be more successful than you have been. This may give rise to a rather bittersweet feeling. All of this contributes to forcing you to confront your own age and heighten the feeling that time is running out and that you had best get on with the job of living and make your mark on the world—now.

Another normal life event that figures in all of this may have to do with the demands on your finances. While you are probably making more money than you have before, you begin to question whether it is enough, whether you will earn more in the future, and whether you will have enough for retirement. If you have teenagers in a college or university, or getting married and starting their own households, you know only too well how much money it takes to help them out, pay for their tuition, or buy them that living room chair. At the same time, you may be feeling that you have worked hard for your money and that it's time *you* started to enjoy the fruits of your labours. What about *your* lifestyle? Isn't it time you bought that luxury car instead of putting up with the old heap? You have always wanted a cottage and if you don't get it now, will you have enough time left to enjoy it?

Another concern that begins to plague some middle-aged workers is the question of retirement. Will there be enough money to enable you to live the way you want to live? How do you want to live? Where will you live? What will you do? Some people prefer to bury their heads in the sand and ignore these questions in the hopes that they will go away, or in the belief that "someone" out there will take care of them in their hour of need. More realistic thinkers know that it *isn't* too early to start thinking along these lines. Besides, their parents won't be there to help them anymore; *they* are the older generation now.

As if this wasn't enough, there may be some things happening with your spouse that can add fuel to the fire. If you are a married male, your wife may already be involved in or about to start her own career. It could well be that just as you are thinking that your career and earning power have peaked, hers is starting to climb. Again, this can be bittersweet. You may be pleased for her, but how will you feel about not being the major breadwinner? If you are a married woman, you may be finding a new and exciting role in life just when your husband seems to be slowing down. You want to get out, meet new people and do things while he wants to come home and relax.

If you are having a mid-career crisis, what can you do about it? The first is to be aware of what is happening and understand that neither the process nor your feelings are unusual. Next, take responsibility for dealing with it. It won't go away and it won't get better by itself. You have to *do* something and deal with the situation. Finally, you must learn how to cope with the crisis. The last is the hardest.

Having your crisis may be the best thing that ever happened to you. Many have found that successful resolutions led to a more enjoyable job, a better lifestyle, new careers, and greater happiness. It's your crisis and you can make out of it what you want.

6. *Men and Women at Mid-Life*

At middle-age both men and women are actually at the apex of their lives. However, as the term suggests, this is a transition point and having reached the top, so to speak, the time after this point is directed towards the end of life. We can look at each of the issues that are pertinent to the person at mid-life, but you will quickly note that we seem to know far more about men and their experiences than we do about women. It's a moot point as to whether this is a result of some sort of sexism among researchers who study these things or not, but I can assure you that I am merely reporting what little we seem to know at this point.

Health—Neither sex suddenly has health problems on achieving the age of 40, but each will notice a general physical decline, a change in body shape and a lessening of energy levels at times. Fat deposits begin to appear in unwanted places, the skin begins to lose some of its elasticity, arthritis may threaten as does osteoporosis for women. Each sex begins to monitor their weight more often and there is a rise in interest in dieting and exercise. Sometimes this ends just at the interest stage and nothing further is actually done about it.

Women experience the additional phenomenon of menopause, a felt loss of attractiveness and a realization that they can no longer bear children. We are just now beginning to focus attention on menopause, a natural outcome of the fact that our population is middle-aged and going through this event. Unfortunately, we still don't know enough about this change. But we do know that it can start as early as in the 30s and lasts until the late 50s with the average age being around 50. There is disagreement about just what is and is not normal during this time and what can or should be done about it. The only symptom that seems indisputable is that of hot flashes and night sweats. We know that hormonal changes are taking place, but the role of estrogen replacement therapy and the dangers of increased cancer risk is still controversial.

Mortality—Men and women both confront their mortality at this stage and as Neugarten says, their focus switches from "time since birth" to "time left to live."

Self-Assessment—This is probably the major undertaking for most middle-aged people. It's more than simply a time when they examine their lives to see where they are; it also involves coming to terms with life's contradictions. In early adulthood, one strives for goals that are pretty well defined, but now the older, wiser person sees that there are certain shades of gray and that things aren't as black and white or as simple as they used to seem.

Sex roles—An interesting thing takes place here that has been observed time and time again. Men at middle-age tend to let go of some of the traditional male traits like aggression and competitiveness and to allow the feminine traits of nurturing, caring, and sympathetic understanding to come to the fore. On the other hand, women become more assertive and seek increased independence.

Generativity—Both sexes accept responsibility for the future generation and this is not restricted to one's offspring. It can also include protégés, younger adults in general, and serving as a mentor for a less experienced person.

Work—This is an extremely important factor in a person's identity. For the man, work provides not only a source of income, but a kind of yardstick (should we say meterstick now) against which he measures his progress. However, most men's careers have reached a plateau at this time and this creates a sort of no-win situation for them. If they have not achieved all that they wanted or have not progressed as far as they had wished, is there enough time and energy to complete the task? If they have achieved what they set out to do, did they set their sights high enough? Should they have done more? Is this all there is?

On the other hand, women are experiencing a new and unprecedented interest in careers and this comes at a time when the children are no longer dependent and there is more time to get involved in a business. Not only are women seeking careers, they are starting businesses of their own. In fact, they are starting them four times faster than men and are twice as successful. This brings its own set of problems though, as you'll see in Chapter Eight. There may be a role reversal here as a woman's career or business takes off, just as her husband's plateaus or begins to decline.

Family—The events that take place around them have an impact at home. Mothers are no longer nurturing small children and find that they have more time for their own interests. The couple's mutual concern with child care now turns to a mutual interest in each other. Hence the roles of mother and father revert to that of wife and husband. The lessening of family demands on the wife often means that she is free to explore new ventures such as a business, or a career, or returning to school. Twenty years ago the presence of a mature student (the euphemism for a middle- aged person) in my class was a rarity. Now my 20-year-old students complain that they are outnumbered by older students who have more life experiences than they have.

Social relationships—This is a very short section because we just haven't got much information about this topic for middle-aged people. We know that women have and maintain more intimate relationships and more and closer same sex friends than do men. This seems to be a function of how we are socialized as children. The only other thing we can say with any degree of accuracy is that regardless of sex, people who have achieved social fulfillment and are most socially active are less stressed than those who are neither fulfilled nor active.

7. The Sandwiched Generation

For the first time in history, middle-aged couples are caught in a social trend called the sandwiched generation. They have children of their own and aging parents who are or are likely to be, dependent upon them. Hence these people are squeezed between their obligations to their own offspring and to their parents who raised them. The person who typically feels the brunt of these pressures is the woman. While the traditional female role of primary caregiver is evolving to include men, it is still that case that women undertake most of the responsibility of caring for children and aging parents. As an added problem today, the typical sandwiched woman is a working mother with children of her own and a full time job.

The pressures on these people can be extreme and while there are some who say that this isn't the problem that it's made out to be, just ask any woman who finds herself caught between these two generations. Those who claim that it isn't a severe problem reason that the middle-aged woman is at the peak of her health and energy, has money to spare because she is part of a dual income family and besides, our parents are living longer and are healthier longer. Most sandwiched women don't agree with this view.

The facts speak for themselves. For the first time in history, middle-aged people have more parents than children. Put another way, it's quite likely that a couple will have four parents between them but they won't have four children of their own. Couple this with the fact that it makes no difference whether the ailing parents are your parents or your in-laws, the woman still finds herself caring for them and the responsibilities can be significant. In fact, it is likely that middle-aged women today will spend an average of 17 years caring for their children and 18 years caring for aging parents. In the United States 18% of the elderly population already live with an adult child and in both the USA and Canada, only 5% of the elderly live in nursing homes. The situation will only worsen since the current generation is delaying childrearing until their 30s and beyond. This means that their parents will likely be well past middle-age and that the younger generation will have young children at home when their parents need them. Couple this with the increased mobility of our families and it is probable that many sandwiched caregivers will find themselves trying to care for parents who do not even live in the same city.

The strains on the sandwiched generation can be very serious. There are financial demands, housing demands, and time demands. Most families cannot afford to put the parents in retirement or nursing homes unless they have insurance plans to cover this. Usually this means finding room in one's own home and sharing the care responsibilities among the rest of the family members. The time demands seem to fall mostly on the women and this has already surfaced as a significant problem for North American businesses as employees take time off to care for sick parents or take them to doctors. A recent Canadian study found that absenteeism for family reasons has increased by 100% in the last decade and 37% of that increase is the result of employees needing to care for aging relatives.

In addition to these strains, there are also psychological pressures on the caregivers. They suffer from elevated levels of guilt and anxiety as they worry about whether they are providing both their parents and their immediate family members with the attention they need. Some industries have recognized the need to assist the caregivers and are offering counseling. A few progressive firms are setting up elder care centers in the workplace similar to child care centers. Unfortunately, some companies are establishing "daughter" streams for career women who find that they must put their career advancement on hold while they care for their parents. Consequently, there is often more relief than grief when the ailing parents die.

We'll deal with more social trends in Chapter Eight, but this is one that pertains especially to middle-aged people. It is also one that will only get more serious as our population ages and our health care systems come under more pressure.

8. *The Hallmarks of Well-being*

Gail Sheehy did a study a few years ago in which she identified a number of women who she felt were good examples of people who had well rounded, successful lives. She called these people (and her book) "Pathfinders." In the process of her study she asked each of her subjects how they knew when they were happy and fulfilled. She compiled their responses into the following ten hallmarks of well-being. Neither she nor I make any claim that they apply equally well to both women and men, but I think you'll find them interesting to say the least. How many apply to you?

1. My life has meaning and direction.
2. I have experienced one or more important transitions in my adult years and have handled these transitions in an unusual, personal, or creative way.
3. I rarely feel disappointed or cheated by life.
4. I have already attained several of the long-term goals that are important to me.
5. I am pleased with my personal growth and development.
6. I am in love; my partner and I love mutually.
7. I have many friends.
8. I am a cheerful person.
9. I am not thin-skinned or sensitive to criticism.
10. I have no major fears.

9. *Where to Go for More Information*

Baruch, G., and J. Brooks-Gunn. (Eds.). *Women in Midlife.* New York: Plenum. 1985.

Baruch, G. K. and R. Barnett. (1986). "Role Quality, Multiple Role Involvement, and Psychological Well-Being in Midlife Women." *Journal of Personality and Social Psychology. 51.* p. 578–85.

Brammer, L. P. Nolen and M. Pratt. *Joys and Challenges of Middle-age.* Chicago: Nelson-Hall. 1982.

Falkenberg, L. and M. Monachello. "Dual career and Dual-Income families: Do They Have Different Needs?" *Journal of Business Ethics.* 1990, *9.* p. 339–51.

Golan, N. *The Perilous Bridge*. New York: Free Press. 1986.

Grambs, J. D. *Women Over Forty*. (rev. ed.). New York: Springer. 1989.

Hepworth, M. and M. Featherston. *Surviving Middle-Age*. Oxford: Basil Blackwell. 1982.

Hunter, S.,and M. Sundel. (Eds.). *Mid-life Myths*. Newbury Park, CA: Sage. 1989.

Neugarten, B. L. (ed). *Middle-Age and Aging*. Chicago: University of Chicago Press. 1968.

Neugarten, B. L. "Must Everything Be a Midlife Crisis?" *Prime Time*. Feb., 1980.

Segell, M. "The American Man in Transition." *American Health*. January-February, 1989. p. 59–61.

Sheehy, G. *Pathfinders*. New York: Morrow. 1981.

Sherman, E. *Meaning in Mid-life Transitions*. Albany: State University of New York Press. 1987.

Tamir, L. M. "Men at Middle-Age." *Annals of the American Academy of Political and Social Science*. Nov., 1982. *464*. 47–56.

Tamir, L.M. *Men in Their Forties*. New York: Springer. 1982.

"Who's Afraid of Middle-Age?" *The Royal Bank Monthly Letter*. Oct., 1979, *60*, 10.

chapter 6

Late Adulthood

Life would be infinitely happier if we could only be born at the age of eighty and gradually approach eighteen.

—Mark Twain

One of the most interesting things about studying this period is that we don't really have very good guidelines about when it starts or what to call it. As more of our population gets older, lives longer, and is healthier at their ages than their parents, the old terms of "senior citizen," the "golden age," "retirees," etc,. no longer seem appropriate. Neugarten has suggested such terms as "the young old" and "the old old," but these haven't caught on. The problem is that we glorify youth in our society and no one wants to be considered old. Nevertheless, we all get old eventually. As Moms Mabley once said about old age, "You just wake up one morning, and you got it!"

Before we get to the information about this stage, let's put the concept of old age into some perspective. Just how long can you expect to live? Don't confuse lifespan with life expectancy. Lifespan is the maximum number of years a person can live. The truth of the matter is that our bodies don't wear out until about the age of 120, but something else usually gets us before that. Life expectancy is the number of years people born at certain times can expect to live. A person born in North America in 1900 had a life expectancy of 48. At the present time the life expectancy has risen to about 79 for women and 72 for men and the projections are that by 2020, the average life expectancy will have risen to 82 for women and 74 for men. It's intriguing to note that the fastest growing age group are those people over 65 and that we now have more people over 100 alive than at any time in our history.

1. The Developmental Tasks

The list of normal developmental tasks for this period is the shortest one we've seen yet, and that is quite in keeping with this stage in life. Much has been accomplished by now and there are simply not as many things that a person must learn how to do. Some of the things that are part of the normal progression through life at this age are:

1. Adjusting to decreasing physical strength and health—This is normally a gradual development and one that gently creeps up on us.

2. Adjusting to retirement and a reduced income—This is a major adjustment for some people and a serious concern for many.

3. Adjusting to the death of a spouse—On average women outlive their husbands by about 12 years. This means that most women will have to face this adjustment and that they will also have to adjust to life without this partner.

4. Establishing sound relationships with one's own age group— There is some minor controversy over this task. While one must come to terms with one's own age, it doesn't necessarily mean that you have to surround yourself with only people your own age. In fact, if there is any truth to the saying that "You are only as old as you think you are." It may not make sense to confine yourself only to older people.

5. Establishing satisfactory living arrangements—This includes deciding where to live when one is healthy and independent and what to do as one needs more care and attention.

6. Adapting to the loss of friends—This will take place through death, illness, and because they will move away into other living arrangements.

7. Deciding on an appropriate lifestyle and level of social involvement—This includes determining whether one will continue to be an active participant in one's society, or whether to disengage from the world. Since we have become an age-irrelevant society, it is now more likely that older people will act as old as they feel and refuse to retire to the rocking chair.

> *Man weeps to think that he will die so soon; woman, that she was born so long ago.*
>
> —H. L. Mencken

2. How are Our Attitudes Towards Aging and the Aged Changing?

Before we can answer this, we must look at some of the prevalent attitudes and use them as a sort of benchmark against which to measure changes. I always start this unit with my classes by giving them a short "Attitudes Towards Aging" test. Here is a shortened version of it. Answer each question True or False.

T	F	1.	Most couples in their 60s no longer enjoy sex.
T	F	2.	As people age, they think more about the past than about the future.
T	F	3.	Older people are less likely to be able to adapt to changes.
T	F	4.	Life satisfaction declines as one gets older.
T	F	5.	Depression is a common affliction for older people.
T	F	6.	Older people start going to church more regularly.

Well, how did you do? It may surprise you to learn that ALL of the answers are false. If you marked even one "true" you are unfortunately like many other people in our society in that you have inappropriate and incorrect information about the elderly.

There are some good reasons for this and it has to do with the fact that few people who aren't old have much contact with older people. Grandparents used to be the best known old people for us, but they may live miles away now and you may not see them very often. If you are part of a reconstituted family (formerly married people who have remarried), the grandparents may have become lost in the shuffle. It also used to be the case that our communities were more open and we all knew older people who lived on our street quite well. Since this has changed, we now get our information about older people from the media, the TV programs we watch, and the books we read. Up to now, the media has been one of the least accurate places to get accurate information about the elderly.

Old is not a four letter word, but many people act as if it was and all of us, regardless of our interest in the elderly are infected by ageism, the negative stereotyping of the elderly resulting in prejudice and discrimination against older people. It's bad enough that society in general subscribes to erroneous views about the elderly, and even worse that the elderly themselves may accept them. However, before we can attempt to remedy the situation, we must understand why it is happening, where it occurs and what effects it has on us.

Ageism isn't really new, but it is becoming more widespread as our society has fewer face-to-face experiences with the elderly. Years ago, in the western world, it was common to have an extended family comprised of several generations living under one roof. This has changed and with the added factors of greater family mobility, divorces, reconstituted families (previously divorced partners marrying) and smaller family units, we simply don't have as much contact with the elderly as before. This is especially true for children who may see their grandparents on very few occasions if at all.

Where then do we see older people and how do we learn about them? It seems that the greatest source of information is via the media; television, advertising, books, magazines, newspapers, and anything but real people. Unfortunately, much of this information is biased, stereotyped and just plain wrong.

Studies of how the elderly are portrayed have found that it was typical for them to be shown as ill, tired, mentally slower, forgetful, unable to learn new ideas, isolated, and unhappy. Ageism is unfortunately all too common in the general population and even in the ranks of those who deal directly with the elderly.

Language is often used to perpetuate ageism. There are two forms of discrimination in language; distortion which involves attributing negative characteristics (such as ill or unhappy) to the elderly and degradation in which the elderly are portrayed as inferior or obnoxious (stupid old men, interfering old women). We also discriminate against the elderly by means of exclusion and subordination. In the first case, we simply do not show the elderly as part of our normal world and in the second case, when we do show them, we relegate them to unimportant, subservient roles.

The danger here is that once we learn these ageist attitudes, it is very hard to correct them. Yet our attitudes are formed very early in life. Children as young as six have generally unfavourable feelings about the elderly. Studies have shown that third grade children (about 9 years old) have more positive feelings about young as opposed to older adults and by the age of eight, most children have already formulated their ideas and attitudes about being old. Once these attitudes are set, they are hard to change. They tend to become part of our mind set that govern how we act. The danger is obvious. If we raise a generation of children who have ageist attitudes, they will treat the elderly badly and will pass laws and vote in accordance with their erroneous and stereotypic views.

But just how are these attitudes formed? Let's begin by looking at school texts. Every child is exposed to these, but what messages are they getting about the elderly? I regret to tell you that one of our textbooks teaches that all Canadian senators are past retirement (which is probably true) but it goes on to say that these senators' most active and fruitful years are behind them! Undoubtedly, there are some senators who would challenge this quite heatedly.

Probably the greatest single source of influence when it comes to attitudes is television. Many studies have proven that television is highly effective in transmitting attitudes and in providing role models. Not only is TV watched by most people, we spend an amazing amount of time watching it and of course, the more we watch, the more we are influenced by what we see. One American researcher says that children spend more time watching TV than they do in school. He found that by the age of 16, the average US child will have spent over 15,000 hours in front of a television set. The elderly too watch a great many hours of TV, but what messages are they getting?

There have been several studies of the way the elderly are portrayed on television. I analysed 50 television programs that were the most popular with elementary school aged children and found that the programs were both sexist and ageist. Men are shown as having the most important, most exciting and most fulfilling roles at every age and even though there are more elderly women than elderly men in our society, television shows just the reverse. Hence the elderly are excluded from society and the roles they do have, according to TV, are really quite dreadful. The most popular roles for older women are first as servants and secondly as witches. Older men fare only marginally better and are shown as either retired with nothing much to do or as blue collar workers performing menial jobs. In most cases, if the elderly appear at all, their characters are undeveloped and they are shown as flat, lifeless, depressed, forgetful, and past oriented.

Children probably watch more TV cartoons than any other kind of programs, but here too, television does its worse. Only 11% of TV cartoon characters are older people. The young are portrayed as bright, positive, and energetic, whereas the elderly are shown to be just the opposite.

Adults watching daytime TV dramas aren't treated to any better images. Only 8% of the characters in these programs are elderly and typically those that are shown are not central to the plots or important in any way. The TV message is clear: older people are dull and useless.

Not every child spends all of his or her time in front of a TV. Many of them read books. But again, what messages are they taking in? We studied this as well and found that when we examined more than 500 of the books most often read by elementary aged children, ageism was a prevalent and recurring theme. The elderly comprised only 9% of all the characters and here too, old men outnumbered old women and both were portrayed in negative, stereotypic ways.

But the problem of ageism is more pervasive than just TV and books. It creeps into other facets of our lives. You may be surprised to learn that greeting cards are some of the worst offenders. Birthday cards are often distasteful to the elderly and even when given to the young adult, they carry strong and very negative messages about getting or being old. Consider these examples.

Roses are red, violets are blue.
One thing makes me happy,
I'm younger than you.

Or how about the message contained in this bit of doggerel?

You're at an age when you
should give up one half of your sex life.
Which half will it be?
Talking about it or thinking about it?

People buying and giving cards like these only support and perpetuate ageism. The surprising thing is that the card manufacturers haven't realized how many older people they are offending and how many older people are potential customers.

The good news is that there are many signs that our attitudes may be changing. Take television for instance. A very popular program now in North America is "Golden Girls," a story of three older, single women who are living together in Florida. This is one of the first times that we have seen older people as the main characters in a television series. In the mornings we are often treated to exercise programs featuring nubile young men and women doing strenuous aerobic exercises. A recent addition to this kind of program is one promoting a more gentle type of exercising and featuring a elderly woman as an exercise model.

Even the television advertisements are changing. Bell Telephone shows a delightful ad in which an older but very modern couple, upon hearing that the grandchildren are about to visit, feverishly change themselves and their home into what they obviously feel is the expected, stereotypic view of the elderly. This is an interesting ad in that it shows both how foolish the stereotype is and just how powerful it is in shaping our behaviours.

The same change is taking place in the print media where we see older people as models in catalogues, advertisements, and news features. Our schools too are waking up to the fact that they have a responsibility to educate the next generation that older people are not useless and over the hill. Hence we are seeing better treatment of the elderly in textbooks, teaching units on or about the elderly, an awareness of the aging of our populations, and a new interest in gerontology, especially at the universities, especially at the post-graduate levels. All of these things are natural outcomes of the growth of the numbers of elderly and their refusal to be discriminated against and treated as second class citizens. However, we have a long way to go before we can overcome the ageism which already exists and which affects each of us to some degree.

There are five challenges to meet.

1. We should examine our own biases and beliefs and see to what extent we have unconsciously allowed ageism to influence our views and behaviours.

2. We should make a conscious effort to accentuate the positive instead of the negative aspects of getting older. Remember that

Picasso was still painting at 91, Michelangelo was sculpting at 90, Vivaldi wrote Falstaff at 80, Pablo Casals was playing in his 90s and Churchill was Prime Minister at 81. The models are there if we care to look for them.

3. Try to extinguish the negatives. Being aware of what is wrong is a start, but we must also take steps to eliminate ageism and to prevent its imposition on others. This may mean that you will have to stand up and be counted and that you will have to speak out when you see examples of ageism, to bring people up short and point out where they are wrong and why.

4. Avoid making ageist remarks yourself, buying ageist greeting cards, or giving your grandchildren books that contain ageist stereotypes. Bring the issue of ageism to the attention of your colleagues. If you want to see real action, write the manufacturers of products that are advertised in an ageist manner telling them what you think of their methods. The fear of losing customers can be more effective in changing behaviours than anything else you can try.

5. Finally, remember that "old" is not a four letter word. Instead, recall that most elderly people are healthy, hearty, and happy. To treat them or think about them as anything else does us all injustice.

3. Three Theories on Aging

Since our social scientists are rather new at this business of studying aging and how older people fit into their society and vice versa, we have developed only three major theories about how all of this works. Let's take each of them in the order in which they were proposed. As you read about them, think of some elderly people you know and decide whether these theories adequately explain their interactions with society.

The Three Theories on Aging

1. The Disengagement Theory
2. The Activity Theory
3. The Social Breakdown or Social
   Reconstruction Theory

---

1. The Disengagement Theory—This theory was developed by Cumming and Henry in 1961. According to their thinking, as older people gradually slow down, they withdraw or disengage from their society. However, society also disengages itself from the older people too. The elderly are more and more preoccupied with themselves, take less and less interest in the world around them, and are less emotionally involved with people. Cumming and Henry postulated that this kind of disengagement was needed in order for the elderly to achieve satisfaction in later life.

This theory has been criticized for some time now since it simply doesn't seem to hold true for many people and it can't be used to explain why some elderly are still active, and happy at being active. According to the disengagement theory, active elderly people really don't want to be that way and ought to be depressed about it. That just doesn't happen.

2. The Activity Theory—The activity theory was developed by Neugarten and her colleagues. They looked at the relationship between activity and general life satisfaction and found that there was a positive relationship between them. That is, the more active old people were, the higher their satisfaction with life. Of course, not everyone is equally active, or active in the same way so the researchers also developed a refinement of the theory to account for this. They suggested that there were four different categories of active types: integrated, armour-de-

fended, passive-dependent, and unintegrated. The integrated people were those who were very involved in their world and who readily engaged in a myriad of activities. The armour-defended types were those who were active, but who were active in ways that were similar to the ways they were involved when they were middle-aged adults. That is, they were active while sort of resisting old age. The passive-dependent people were not as active as either of the first two groups and often were somewhat passive and had to be dragged into an activity. The unintegrated types are exactly what they seem to be. They aren't interested, organized, or very involved in any activities. You probably won't be very surprised to learn that the people who had the highest scores on life satisfaction were the most active ones, the integrated and armored-defended types. The least active type, passive-dependent, and unintegrated were the least satisfied. The conclusion is that it is better to be active and involved in one's world. Satisfaction with life diminishes as one withdraws from the world or has an important role taken away. This can occur when one retires or is put into a nursing or retirement home.

3. The Social Breakdown or Social Reconstruction Theory—This is the latest and most promising theory. Developed by Kuypers and Bengstom in 1973, this theory takes the position that one of the prime factors in the promotion of aging is a negative self-concept and negative feedback from other people and society in general about being old. The idea is that if we actually believe that we are old, useless, and incompetent, we are setting up a self-fulfilling prophecy and we will begin to act this way. This theory puts the responsibility for successful aging at the feet of both the elderly themselves and the people who make up their society. The only way to prevent the social breakdown process is to educate society and the elderly themselves about the aging process, to eliminate ageism, and to present more positive images of the elderly. To some extent this

has begun with some of the television programs and movies that feature older people in more positive roles, but we still have a long way to go.

4. The Effect of Separation on Older Adults

There are two major kinds of separations that are particularly difficult for people, especially older adults. Both involve the loss of a spouse. Up to fairly recently, the main cause of such a loss was through death, but older people are also divorcing in greater numbers and there is reason to believe that this is more difficult for them than for younger people. I'll deal with the affects of both losses in this section, but I am going to focus on what happens in a divorce. You will find more information on widows and widowhood in the next section.

For years and years, divorce among older adults who had been married for a long period of time was almost unheard of. However, this has changed and many long term marriages are dissolving. In fact, the number of divorces among people 65 years of age and over more than doubled from 1960 to 1979 and this trend is continuing. Now, don't be alarmed by this statistic because it is very hard to get an accurate perception of the problem, and figures can be read in many different ways. Suffice to say that this is a trend, that divorce in later years is increasing and that our best estimates are that if the trend continues, one woman in eight will have her first marriage end in divorce after she reaches the age of 40.

But what does this do to people and who copes best? It doesn't matter whether an individual suffers a loss of a spouse through death or divorce, a person still has to adjust to the loss and rearrange their life. Emotional ties with the spouse must be broken, the role of wife or husband must be abandoned and daily routines must be changed. Everyone seems to go through three phases: separation, a transitional period, and adaptation and adjustment.

Compared with younger adults, older people going through these phases seem to have a harder time of it. Older people have greater morale problems. Older men who divorce are significantly less happy than women going through the same event, and recently separated men report more feelings of a lack of well being than women. On the other hand, the women seem to have more emotional problems. In addition, older people of both sexes have a harder time fitting back into society than do their younger counterparts. While this is hard for anyone at any age, the over 50 age group have the most difficult time. The same thing applies to the disruption of their lives in general. Those over 50 suffer the most disruption, but women suffer less in this regard than do men. Older women seem to have fewer options open to them than do the men, but regardless of sex, all of these negative effects of a loss increase with age.

5. The Effects of The Death of a Spouse

While I'm going to deal with both widows and widowers in this section, I'm going to concentrate on widows because there are so many of them in comparison with widowers. This is an important topic for anyone studying the lifespan and for people in general because most women today are simply not prepared for the death of their spouse. At the present time in North America, there are far more widows that widowers. In Canada and the USA almost every other woman over the age of 65 is a widow. Widows currently outnumber widowers by a factor of about 3 to 1. This means that a woman is likely to spend as much time as a widow as she did raising children. Coupled with the reality that the average widow may live another 20 years after her husband's death, you can see the magnitude of the problem. But just what are the problems that widows and widowers face?

Many researchers have studied people who have lost a spouse and the findings are all quite similar. But before we turn to these, let me point out that we are concentrating here on the older widow and widowers. Unfortunately, it is possible to lose a spouse at any age and about 13% of all women over 18 are or have been widows. Regardless of the age, the death of a spouse is characterized by grief, bereavement, a sudden change in roles, and a host of adjustments. I'll have more to say about how to cope or help someone cope later on in Chapter Seven, but for now, let's look at the typical kinds of problems widows and widowers experience.

Older women certainly have more problems than older men especially when it comes to maintaining their homes and their health. Unless they are unusually handy with tools and have the physical strength and stamina required, home repair may be beyond their capabilities. There is quite a bit of truth in the definition of a homeowner as, "A person frequently seen leaving the hardware store." The current cohort of older widows is a group of women who were raised in another generation where the traditional sex roles were much stronger than they are today, but regardless of whether the widows in the next generation will differ or not, today's widows need to rely on someone else to perform regular home maintenance. Consequently, many widows just aren't comfortable living alone and seek the assistance of, you guessed it, their daughters and daughters-in-law to help them organize home maintenance.

Older men as widowers who are not comfortable living alone tend to remarry. It is much easier for them to do this since there are relatively few of them and they may be viewed as a sought after commodity. Most men of this generation are used to being married and having someone looking after their needs, so they are not at all adverse to remarrying. This is not meant to denigrate such marriages. I well remember my father-in-law bringing an older widower friend home after one of my son's baptisms where he met a "courtesy aunt" who was the same age and who had never been married. You can guess what happened. This was a particularly happy marriage for them and a delight for all of us.

The other major problems of widowed persons involves coming to terms with the reality that the spouse has died and the fear of what life will be like without them. Loneliness is a severe difficulty for more than half of all widows and somewhat less of a problem for widowers. This seems to hit hardest at meal times, at night, and when shopping or going to social events. Some widows find it very hard to make decisions alone and even when they do, are anxious about whether the decision has been the correct one. Another major change is that of one's identity and role in society. The survivor is no longer a husband or a wife, but must carve out a new identity as a widow or widower. Initially, there is a tendency to hold on to the old roles and the old friends. However, the widow or widower soon finds that they are a "fifth wheel" in a couple-oriented society and their social circle may not be a very welcome or comfortable place anymore. The time needed to adjust to the death of a spouse varies from person to person, but it may take 2 to 3 years before the survivors have worked through their grief, acknowledged that life is no longer the same and adjusted to a new role.

6. *Retirement*

It has been observed that aging isn't so bad when one considers the alternative, but this can't be applied to the retirement process. We mustn't forget that retirement is not a normal or universal stage in the life cycle. Rather, it is an invention of society and one that has been most widely available to industrialized nations only in the past three decades. The thing to remember about retirement is that while it will undoubtedly become a normal experience of most elderly people, it seems to imply that one has some control over one's future. This isn't necessarily true at all.

When retirement first appeared, it was promoted as a time of well deserved rest, a golden age of leisure and a generally great experience for people. This was certainly the image that business, industry, and insurance companies wanted to promote. At the same time, general folk wisdom and the media tended to perpetuate myths about retirement and what happened to people after they retire. Consequently, there are innumerable stories about people who retire and then either wither away and die through boredom or disease, or drive their spouses crazy by taking up hare brained ideas such as selling the family home and traveling the world in a camping van or sailboat. All of these stories follow a similar plot. The retiree makes bad decisions, loses money, fails to find happiness, dies, and his or her spouse follows them to the grave six months later. These stories are fallacious and are not borne out by what actually happens to most people.

But before we get to the truth, it is worthwhile knowing how these myths get started and how they are perpetuated. Gerstl reviewed hundreds of magazines, business publications, and specialized publications which carried articles about retirement. He found that over the last 40 years, only half of the articles presented anything close to a positive view of retirement, and that 40% of them depicted retirement as something that is never as satisfying as work, that it is like being put out to pasture, and that it is generally negative. Hence it seems that at least up to now, the media have perpetuated erroneous myths about retirement. This will likely change as more and more people retire. But a lasting change will require an attitude in which retirement is seen as not just an absence of work but a new beginning to a period that may last for up to a third of the total lifespan.

Why is retirement a crisis for some people and not for others? What happens to people as they approach retirement and after they are completely retired? Are there predictable stages to retirement? As our population ages and more and more people approach retirement, we are becoming increasingly interested in these and other questions about the entire retirement process.

People generally have very mixed feelings about retirement and tend not to think about it until it is just around the corner. Yet there are now more than 300 Canadians retiring every day of the year and we know that this figure will increase as our population ages. At the present time, we are a middle-aged nation, but in the near future, we will become a "young old" nation. The demographic trend is as follows:

Canadian Data	
Year	Millions over 65
1978	2.1
2000	3.4
2030	6.8

Coupled with this is the fact that more and more people are retiring. In 1900 only 32% of men over 65 had retired. In 1980 80% of the over 65's were retired. The average length of time spent in retirement is now nineteen years (this will change to twenty five years by the year 2000).

Given these figures, it is astounding that so few people are preparing for their retirement and that so few companies are taking any interest in their employees' future well-being. Anyone who thinks about the future has to be concerned about how they will cope for approximately one quarter of their lifespan.

Regardless of who you are—your sex, your job, your position, your financial situation, or even how prepared you think you may be for it—retirement is a stressful transition that may trigger unexpected results. Up to now, we have primarily thought of retirees as males, but this picture is rapidly changing as more career women (and often single women) retire. They, too, tend to have the same reactions as men, plus a few wrinkles of their own. Having studied thousands of retirees, we can predict what the normal reactions will be.

First, one leaves work and goes through a period of missing one's colleagues. This is followed by an outward acceptance of retirement and a sort of *honeymoon* time when everything looks great. Next the retiree feels some *anger and resentment* at being rejected by his or her firm and by society in general. After a while, this is replaced by the opposite view and on is *thankful* for being released from the rat race, the daily grind and the nine-to-five routine. This stage is followed by an attitude of *determined enjoyment;* the retiree decides to enjoy the years to come no matter what. Unfortunately, he or she may not know how to make this happen.

Next comes an *adjustment* phase in which the recent retiree tries to live with new decisions, a new lifestyle, new interests and new demands. Often this is also a time when the retiree drives his or her spouse mad, becomes an aimless irritant, and dabbles in a variety of short-lived hobbies, interests or hare-brained schemes.

This stage usually has a happy ending with the retiree finally making the transitions and learning how to relax and enjoy life. For some, however, the new interests and activities aren't as enjoyable as the old job and a state of perpetual wistfulness sets in resulting in discontent and unhappiness.

The good news is that most people are able eventually to make all the transitions and to live with retirement. In fact 75% adjust and adjust well. However, this process takes time and of course there are the 25% for whom it never takes place. All of this makes a very strong argument for sound, early, pre-retirement planning. This is especially true for anyone who wishes to live on anything more than their company pension and the old age pension. Financial planning requires at least a 15-year head start if you want to build a decent nest egg.

There are a variety of psychological phases, pressures and events that hit at retirement. We know how to head off the worst of these and how to cope with the remainder. There are certain problems and concerns which apply to most retirees. The most common problems and the percentage of retirees who had them is shown below.

Common Problems	
Money	64%
Nostalgia	49%
Family	48%
Boredom	37%
Transportation	32%
Health	31%
Loneliness	29%
Uselessness	26%
Housing	23%
Not having enough to do	16%

How can you make the necessary adjustments and avoid these problems? Follow these steps. They will enable you to cope with retirement faster and more easily.

1. Anticipate, plan and prepare for your retirement. Start at least 15-years before you retire and get expert help and advice.

2. Be prepared to face the reality that you will retire. Those who deny that it has happened or try to ignore it, won't be successful.

3. Take responsibility for your life after retirement. Don't rely on your spouse to keep you occupied, or the adult recreation director to think up new interests for you.

4. Be interested in people. People-oriented persons are much more likely to adjust faster and better than whose who avoid social contacts.

5. Cultivate a variety of interests. The more you have, the better.

6. Look to the future. Don't take the attitude that its all over for you and downhill from here on in. This kind of thinking makes it so.

7. Maintain your health and fitness. These two factors are absolutely vital to the success of everything else.

8. Keep in touch with old friends and make new ones. Old friends are like wine, they generally improve with age, but it is nice to sample something different once and a while.

9. Take care of your personal appearance. Don't fall into the trap of dressing in old, out-of-date clothing, or salvation army rejects unless you are cleaning out the septic tank. You feel good when you look good.

10. Adapt to new situations and learn to welcome change. Change is inevitable and kicking against it won't prevent it. Learn to "go with the flow."

11. Last of all, learn to relax and enjoy life. This sounds easy, but too many hard drivers have never mastered this skill. You've earned your retirement, so enjoy it.

Is retirement a crisis? It's really up to you. It only becomes a crisis if you let it. But the time is now to take steps to prepare for what should be a most pleasant time.

7. *Death, Dying, and the Grief Process*

It has often been said that we are a death denying society. It's certainly true. These days one can talk about almost anything in front of almost anybody. We think nothing of openly discussing the most private things, things that our parents and earlier generations would never have talked about to anyone. However, when it comes to death, we all shy away from it; try to ignore it, and are very awkward when we do have to confront it. While it is true that everyone will die eventually, we prefer *not* to think about this and if we do have to talk about it, we speak in euphemisms such as "passed away", "gone to their reward," etc.

The reasons why we are this way have a lot to do with how we were raised, our experiences, beliefs, and the way life and death are presented in the media. One of our greatest fears is that of the unknown and this is one of the reasons we fear death. This is where the strength of your religious convictions play a part in lessening that fear. Death holds fewer terrors for the person who firmly believes in a life hereafter. But our view of death is certainly shaped by the media and what we see around us. The symbolism of death has been used time and time again to terrorize us in ghost stories and horror movies. The image of death as portrayed at Halloween parties with ghost and skeleton costumes, and our images of spooky graveyards and fearsome monsters returning from the dead all contribute to our fear. Coupled with this is our tendency to present death as evil so it is no wonder that we have this negative attitude about death. In fact, the whole idea of death being negative is common in our society, and it has been said that North Americans view death as a failure.

It wasn't always this way. We have lost our respect and familiarity with death. Where it once was a common occurrence that took place in public view, we now treat death as something we should hide and as something that is unnatural. Only a few generations ago, people died at home and were often either buried from the home or at least lay there for a few days before the actual burial. This gave everyone, including children, first hand experience with death in a familiar setting. This made it seem more natural and took a great deal of the terror away.

I remember my grandfather dying at home and lying in the front room for a few days while people came to pay their respects. The family life continued on around him and even as a young boy, I felt that it was right that he be there in his house with the rest of the family. This was quite different from my father's death which took place out of our sight in a sterile hospital. After he died, he was taken to a funeral home where we were told what to do and when to do it. This kind of dying makes it seem remote and institutionalized and it contributes to our fears.

Grief is a normal reaction at a time of death, but remember that grief can also occur at other times. In fact, grief normally follows the loss of anything that is important to a person. Consequently, grief reactions are experienced many times over the lifespan and in varying degrees of intensity. Grief is a normal part of living. Our reactions to it follow a set pattern and we must go through the grief process before we can return to a normal state.

The intensity and duration of our reactions to grief depend on our reaction to the particular loss we are experiencing and our experience with grief. Three things are usually present when a grief reaction takes place: loss, value, and impact. There is a loss, the thing that is lost is valuable and one has an emotional reaction. The things that determine the effect that grief will have on a person are the intensity of the motions one feels, the value one attaches to the loss, and the perception that one has of the effect that this loss will have on one's life. While it is easy to see that one will experience grief when a loved one dies, it is also true that grief can also be experienced at retirement, the end of a personal relationship, when one's children leave home, or when there is a separation or a divorce. In fact, divorce has been called the little death, for just this reason.

The grief process may take a long or a short period of time, but everyone works through the process in their own way, with or without help. Our knowledge of the stages that people go through in the grief process date back to the work that Linderman did while working with the survivors of the disastrous fire at the Coconut Grove nightclub in the 1940s. He suggested that people go through nine stages in dealing with their grief.

Linderman's Nine Stages of Grief
1. Shock
2. Emotional Response
3. Isolation
4. Physical Symptoms
5. Panic
6. Guilt
7. Anger
8. Reaching Out
9. Reenter Life

---

1. Shock—This is a natural reaction to a serious situation. It is the way we defend ourselves from the reality of what has happened by using a kind of temporary anesthesia. Normally, this only lasts for a short period of time before reality asserts itself and we face up to what has actually occurred. Prolonged escape is dangerous.

2. Emotional Response—It is only human to express emotions and this is the stage where that occurs. Our emotions may be positive or negative, socially acceptable or unacceptable. Much will depend on the person, the situation, and the culture. Some people cry, some maintain a stiff upper lip and try to not show any motion, while in some situations and some cultures, people wail and become hysterical.

3. Isolation—This is the stage at which a person feels depressed and isolated from the normal world. Nothing seems to be the

way it used to be. People may also feel that no one completely understands what they are feeling or going through and that they are very much alone in their grief.

4. Physical Symptoms—Because of the increased stress levels, all of the normal stress reactions may appear and some of them may be extreme. Hence, it is not uncommon to have eating and sleeping disorders, emotional highs and lows, irritability, physical ailments, stomach and digestive upsets, etc.

5. Panic—When the grief becomes overwhelming, it is easy to feel overwhelmed and that things (including you) are out of control. This can lead to a feeling of panic and an inability to think rationally.

6. Guilt—People who are experiencing grief often feel guilty about things they have done, or failed to do or even the way they are reacting to their loss. They may wish they had done something to prevent or alleviate the loss; that they had said something to the person who has died before they died, or they may regret something they did or said to the person. In many cases, the person who is left behind may be very angry at the person who is gone for leaving them. When the person has died, the survivors may feel guilty that they even harbor these thoughts. Yet this is a normal reaction. I remember my mother being very angry that my father had died and left her alone and then being consumed with guilt that she even thought this about the poor guy.

7. Anger—This too is a normal reaction and a part of the grief process. The anger can be turned towards the person who has died, but it can also be turned towards God for allowing this to occur, or to those who are not experiencing this loss. For example, a widow may feel a kind of resentful anger towards her friends whose husbands have not died. Often this anger is directed towards the doctors, nurses, social service agencies, insurance companies, or anybody else that has had anything to do with the loss.

8. Reaching out—This is the stage in which the survivor reaches out to others in the hope and expectation that they will somehow help them through this painful period. People may make frequent and unreasonable demands on relatives and friends and expect that they will immediately leap to their aid even if it interferes with their own lives. This can cause resentment and anger on the part of both those who are approached for help and the person who is receiving it. Much will depend on the expectations of both parties. How much help is appropriate? There is a tendency in our society to expect and want people to get on with their lives, and we are uncomfortable being around those who don't recover and bounce back quickly. We get impatient with teenagers who have trouble getting over the loss of a relationship and we wish not to be involved with people who are saddened by the loss of a loved one.

9. Reenter Life—This is the finale and culminating stage of grief and the one in which a person makes a recovery. However, experiencing a loss is a transition that changes us and our lives, sometimes in significant and long lasting ways. A person will be changed by the experience and one's life may be quite different than it was before the loss. It's easy to see this in the case of a person whose spouse has died, but it is equally true in cases involving the loss of a pet, graduating from school, a financial setback, or even losing a valued possession.

There is only one thing age can give you, and that is wisdom.

—S.I. Hayakawa.

8. *Where Do You Get More Information*

Bahr, S. J., and E. T. Peterson. (Eds.). *Aging and the Family.* Lexington, MA: Lexington Books. 1989.

Cain, B. S. "Divorce among Elderly Women: A Growing Social Phenomenon." *Social Casework: The Journal of Contemporary Social Work.* Nov., 1988. p. 563–568.

Campbell, S., and P. R. Silverman. *Widower.* New York: Prentice-Hall Press. 1987.

Carey, R. G. "Weathering Widowhood: Problems and Adjustment of the Widowed During the First Year." *OMEGA,* 1979–80, *10,* 2. p. 163+.

Cohen, S. and T. A. Wills. "Stress, Social Support and the Buffering Hypothesis." *Psychological Bulletin.* 1985, 98. p. 310–57.

Delongis, A., J. C. Coyne, G. Dakof, S. Folkman, and R. S. Lazarus. "Relationship of Daily Hassles, Uplifts and Major Life Events to Health Status." *Health Psychology.* Jan., 1982, *1.* p. 119–36.

Essa, Mohsain. "Grief as a Crisis: Psychotherapeutic Interventions with Elderly Bereaved." *American Journal of Psychotherapy.* 1986, *40.* p. 243–51.

"Facing Up to Death." *The Royal Bank Letter.* May/June 1982, *63,* 3.

Farnsworth, J., M. A. Pett, and D. A. Lund. "Predictors of Loss Management and Well-Being in Later Life, Widowhood, and Divorce." *Journal of Family Issues,* March 1989, *10,* 1. p. 102–21.

Halpern, James. *Helping Your Aging Parents.* New York: McGraw Hill. 1987.

Horowitz, A. "Sons and Daughters as Caregivers to Older Parents." *Gerontologist.* Jan, 1985, *25.* p. 612–617.

Kahana, E. F. and H. A. Kiyak. "The Older Woman: Impact of Widowhood and Living Arrangements on Service Needs." *Journal of Gerontological Social Work.* Winter 1980, *3,* 2. p. 17–29.

Kalish, R. A. *Death, Grief and Caring Relationships*. Montery, CA: Brooks/Cole. 1981.

Kubler-Ross, E. *Death, the Final Stage of Life*. Englewood Cliffs, NJ: Prentice Hall. 1973.

Lindemann, E. "Symptomatology and Management of Acute Grief." *American Journal of Psychiatry*. 1944, *101*. p. 141–148.

O'Connor, D. J. and D. M. Wolfe. "On Managing Midlife Transitions in Career and Family." *Human Relations*. 1987, *40*, 12. p. 799–816.

Osterweis, M. "Bereavement and the Elderly." *Aging*. 1985 *348*. p. 8+.

Pallmore, E. B., B. M. Burchett, G. G. Fillenbaum, L. K. George, and L. M. Wallman. *Retirement: Causes and Consequences*. New York: Springer. 1985.

Parkes, C. M. *Bereavement: Studies of Grief in Adult Life*. London: Tavistock Publications. 1972.

Ruple, S. W. "Grief: The Hidden Crisis." *Emotional First Aid*. 1985, *2*, 3. p. 10–15.

Schwartzen-Borden, G. "Grief Work: Prevention and Intervention." *Social Casework: The Journal of Contemporary Social Work*. 1986. p. 499–503.

Silverman, P. R. "Widowhood and Preventative Intervention." *The Family Coordinator*. 1972. *21*, 1. p. 95–102.

Singleton, J. F. "Retirement: Its Effects on the Individual." *Activities, Adaptation and Aging*. Summer 1985, *6*, 4. p. 1–7.

Uhlenberg, P., C. Cooney, and R. Boyd. "Divorce for Women after Midlife." *Journal of Gerontology: Social Sciences* 1990, *45*, 1. S3–11.

chapter 7

Crisis, Defenses and Crisis Intervention

*Psychiatry is the art of teaching
people how to stand on their own feet
while reclining on couches.*

—Shannon Fife

1. Introduction

When unpleasant things happen to people, they unconsciously try to protect themselves from the discomfort and to cope with the situation as best they can. We all do this. But why are some people able to cope while others never seem to be able to handle their problems? Why is it that some folks fall into despair while others survive, adjust, and carry on? How can you help a person who is going through a crisis? That's what this chapter is all about. We'll be looking at what happens during a crisis, how we defend ourselves, how and under what conditions we adjust and what actually occurs during a time of stress.

Before we get to the psychological content, I want to make sure that you understand what we are talking about. We seem to use the term crisis very loosely these days and everyone talks about having a crisis even if all that is wrong with them is a hangnail. Not every problem that you experience is a crisis in the psychological sense of the word. For our purposes here, we will be using crisis to mean a problem that a person cannot handle without the help of someone else. That is, they need someone to assist them to find a solution. They may not be able to handle it because they have never encountered it before, because they don't have the skills to deal with it, or because they are so upset that they can't see how to apply the skills they already possess.

We know quite a bit about crises, what causes them, the normal stages that people go through, what is normal, what is abnormal and most importantly, how to help ourselves and others when a crisis occurs. But keep in mind that none of this is set in concrete. That is, these are models of what can happen and while they are based on studies of what has transpired with thousands of people, not everyone will go through all of the stages in the same ways. Nevertheless, we can anticipate that when faced with what seem to be insurmountable pressures and a situation that they cannot manage alone, people tend to react by withdrawing, feeling helpless, trying to overcontrol some aspect of the situation, keeping it all inside themselves or letting it all go in fits of emotional outbursts. What I want to do here is to help you make some sense out of people's behaviors and to prepare you to be of assistance when these situations happen.

2. What Happens in a Crisis?

Researchers have found that there are four major phases in most crisis situations.

The Four Crisis Phases

1. Shock
2. Denial (defensive retreat)
3. Acknowledgment
4. Adaptation

Let's take an example and go through each phase and see how it works. Imagine this situation. You have borrowed your mother's new sports car (without her permission) and are taking it for a quick joy ride when you suddenly smash into a garbage truck that seemed to appear from nowhere. As you sit in the now crumpled sports car nursing your nose where it bumped against the steering wheel, you feel confused and disoriented. In fact, you are so upset that when the burley truck driver appears to ask if you are OK, you have trouble answering and can't seem to remember your current address. You are not losing your mind. You are simply in a state of shock.

This state seems to pass very quickly, but at almost the same time you enter the second phase (denial or defensive retreat) and are heard to say, "Oh no! This must be a bad dream! Tell me it isn't true!" Again, this is quite normal and you are simply in the stage where you naturally apply the normal defense mechanisms to attempt to shield yourself from the reality of what has happened. This is what is occurring when you hear people say these same things when they are told that a catastrophe has happened. Of course, reality eventually sets in and you have to face the fact that Mom's car is smashed beyond recognition. This part is normal. What is not normal is to continue to pretend that the event hasn't happened. People who get stuck at this stage end up with serious problems. Sometimes this happens when loved ones have been killed and the survivors just can't bring themselves to face the facts.

The third phase of acknowledgment takes place after reality has been reestablished. This is when you admit that the car really is smashed, that you really are in deep trouble and that you had better figure out what to do about it. Now note that while you have faced the facts, you may or may not have any idea about what you should actually do. However, it is at this stage that you either figure out a solution or someone else can assist you. No one will be successful in trying to help you while you are still in a state of shock or while you are in denial.

The fourth and final stage of adaptation occurs sometime after you have decided on and implemented a workable solution. In our example, you may rush home, confess and throw yourself on your mother's mercy. If you are lucky, she'll be so glad that no one was injured, she'll not be mad about the car.

Note that I said that adaptation happens sometime afterwards. Adaptation may occur immediately, or slowly over a period of days, weeks or even years. It all depends on you, your experience with crises and the severity of the event. It usually takes you longer the first time to learn how to adjust and then it will be faster after that. In other words, the second time you smash a car, the more likely it is that your recovery time will be accelerated. However, we know that it may take three years or more to adjust to the death of a spouse.

But I also said that it had to be a workable solution. Getting your friend to help you push Mom's car over the nearest cliff and then pretending that you know nothing about it probably won't work. While this may seem to be an extreme example, it is not very different from the person who simply refuses to admit that some event has occurred and tries to lie their way out of the consequences.

There is much more to these four phases if we consider what happens to a person in terms of the stress they feel, their emotions, view of reality, and ability to think. Let's take each phase in turn and see what can happen.

Shock—This is a period of intense stress since the person sees the event as presenting some kind of threat. Smashing into that garbage truck can certainly be seen as a threat of a loss—your life, Mom's car, your freedom, etc. At this stage, the person sees the situation as overwhelming and may feel anxious, helpless, and even panicky. It is natural that they cannot think clearly and will be unable to organize, plan, or to understand someone else who is trying to reason with them.

Denial—In this phase, the person's subconscious takes over and tries to block out the threat so that the old ways can be maintained. At this point, the person is blocking out reality and engaging in wishful thinking, and using the normal defense mechanisms of denial and repression. Some peculiar things can happen to the emotions at this stage. On the one hand, the person may appear to be indifferent, or they can appear to be in a kind of happy, euphoric state. Sometimes we see this when something serious has happened and the person who is involved gets the giggles. You may remember this happening to you. This makes other people confused as they can't see anything funny in the situation. Of course there isn't anything funny and this is only a nervous reaction. The usual outcome of this sequence is that when the giggler is challenged with, "What are you laughing at? There's nothing funny about this." The giggler's feelings turn to anger and more confusion results.

Acknowledgment—During this phase, reality asserts itself and the person faces up to what has actually happened. However, this causes an increase in stress as the person now has to confront the truth. This can lead to feelings of depression, bitterness, mourning, extreme anxiety and even suicide. It is not unusual, for example, for widows to become suicidal at this point. The thought processes at this stage go through a transition from disorganization at the start of the period to reorganization as the person comes to grips with what has happened.

Adaptation—In the final phase, the person develops a new view of reality, adjusts to a changed situation, establishes an improved and changed sense of self worth and experiences gradually increasing feelings of satisfaction. This may take a long period of time, depending on the seriousness of the crisis event.

Once you know about these four phases, you can analyse what is happening in a crisis, determine the stage a person is in and know what to expect. Try it on this crisis that happened to me. Two weeks after I bought my first sports car (a bright green Triumph), it stalled and I got out, opened the hood and reached under the engine to check a loose wire. A few seconds later, a woman drove into the back of my car at 30 miles an hour, catapulting me and the car about 100 yards down the street. I was furious and after I had extracted myself from the engine, I rushed back to confront her. As I approached, she got out of her car and promptly fainted. When I stopped and looked at myself, I realized that my arm was badly cut and that I was covered with blood, but I didn't feel anything. How would you explain her reaction and mine?

If you said we were both in a state of shock, you would be correct. The interesting thing is that we had different physical reactions. Hers was to faint (the ultimate form of cognitive denial!) while in my case, there was physical shock which numbed me to the pain.

3. Hopson's Cycle of Reactions

People who have studied the reactions that people exhibit when faced with a crisis have found that a common pattern of responses. Hopson suggests that there are seven major changes in one's self esteem from the beginning of a crisis until it ends. You won't have to look very closely to see that these seven factors are very similar to the four crisis phases you read about earlier.

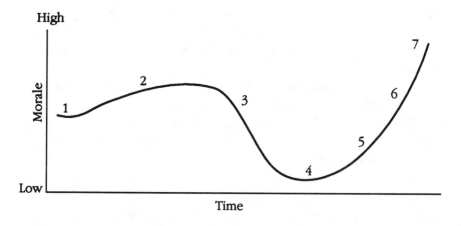

1. Immobilization—This is a sense of being overwhelmed and being unable to plan, organize, think rationally, or understand what is happening.

2. Minimization—This is similar to the phases known as denial.

3. Depression—As reality sets in, people have to face what has happened and the truth may make them anxious, angry, or depressed. In any event, their morale generally drops.

4. Letting Go—This is the beginning of the transition phase and it involves letting go of the attachment one had to the reality, person, object or thing involved in the crisis.

5. Testing—This is another transition phase and one that generally sees the person trying out the changes that he or she must make. It's a bit like experimenting with something before committing oneself to it completely. For example, a divorced person might go out on a date or two to see if this is what they want to do and to explore their feelings about it.

6. Search for meaning—This appears at the end of the experimentation phase. During this phase, the person is trying to understand just what the transition will mean for them and whether he or she will want to commit to it entirely.

7. Internalization—This is the last stage in the transition process. It is similar to the adaptation stage we talked about earlier. At this point, the person has made the transition to a different form of behaviour, or lifestyle, or way of functioning and we can say that the transition is complete.

The interesting thing about Hopson's model is that it shows in greater detail, just how a person's emotions and morale are affected when they go through a crisis or transition.

4. The Factors for Effective Coping

Why is it that some people seem to deal with any situation that crops up, while others are unable to handle even simple problems without falling apart? You will have met both kinds of people in your working and personal relationships and may even have examples of them in your own family. Perhaps if you look closely enough, you will be able to see yourself as either one type or the other. In fact, there is really a bit of both in each of us and even the person that seems calm and unruffled most of the time, can come up against a situation that he or she cannot handle.

You are fortunate if you are or work with the kind of person that is a calm, effective coper. This type of person can respond quickly and easily to situations. He never seems to lose control; he is rational and logical and come, across as being unflappable. At the other extreme, we all know people who seem to come apart at the slightest problem, who lose their cool and react in seemingly irrational ways. In between these two, we find the person who appears to be strong, well adjusted, and capable and then, all of a sudden, something happens that makes them go off the deep end. What is going on here? How does one explain such behaviour?

In reality, the explanation is fairly simple. Psychologists who have studied subjects' reactions to events have learned that there is a pattern to the way they respond and that there are certain characteristics which differentiate between conditions that lead to successful coping and those that bring on full-fledged crises. First of all, let's get one thing straight. It is not the event itself that causes a crisis. It is how one reacts to it that determines whether one can handle it easily, or not at all. My model of the stages and sequence in a crisis looks like this.

A Crisis Flow Chart

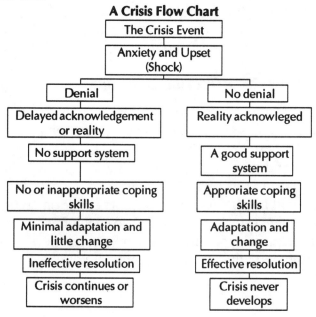

Let's use an ordinary event and see why it leads to a crisis for one person but not for another. For sake of argument, we will consider the event of being fired. Is this a crisis or not? Well, it depends on a variety of factors: you, how you perceive it, whether you have adequate support, and whether you know how to cope. To start, we will follow down the left side of the chart and see how the event does lead to a full scale, humdinger of a problem.

Our victim (let's call him Sam) has just been called into the boss's office and told that he is being fired because of his continuous petty theft of company supplies. Sam's immediate reaction, similar to the scene in the movie "Mr. Mom," is to leap across the desk and try to strangle his boss. After the security guards pull him off and toss him out, Sam goes home and tells his wife what has happened. When she asks why, he tells her that it was because his bosses hated him, had it in for him, and unreasonably objected to him taking home the company computer when they knew full well that he was only using it for office work.

This is the first problem. Sam is using denial as a defense mechanism to avoid confronting his responsibility for what has happened. In psychological terms, he does not have a realistic perception of the event.

At this point, his wife turns on him and yells, "You jerk! You no good bum! I should have listened to my mother. She always said you were a turkey. We have eight kids and your brother to feed and now you go and get yourself fired. Sam, you're a real loser!"

This is the second problem stage. Sam doesn't seem to be getting much support from the home front. By now, he is angry, depressed, and confused. He is embarrassed by being fired and he simply doesn't know what to do or whom to turn to. Rather than let the neighbours think he is unemployed, he drives off each morning as if he was going to work, but in fact, he spends his day hitting the bottle. Things come to a head two months later when he is arrested for drunk driving, he is sent to jail; his wife and children leave him and his house burns down. Now he has a grand scale crisis. Oh, all right. Maybe we did overdo it a little bit, but let's look at what happened.

Sam started drinking because he didn't know what else to do. In other words, he has no repertoire of coping skills. In fact, he regressed to rather primitive behaviour—going straight for his boss's jugular, and his drinking is more denial and escapism. The problem continues and in fact gets worse which is normally the case in such situations.

Now let's take the same event and follow it through to a no-crisis resolution. Our victim this time is a Mehitabel, a single parent who is about to be fired. Mehitabel, (known to her friends as Bel) is called into her boss's office where she is informed that the company is retrenching and her department is being phased out; hence, there are no other positions available for her. Bel is angry and resentful, but she cleans out her desk and heads for home.

That evening she has supper with a friend and explains what has happened and that it is not due to any fault on her part. In other words, she has a realistic perception of what has happened. Having had time to cool down a bit, she tells her friend that she doesn't know what to do, but that she has had it with working for others. She has always wanted to start her own business and she thinks that this might just be the opportune time to do so, if only she knew how to go about it. Bel's friend encourages her in this direction and tells her that she is bright, capable, hardworking, a fantastic computer analyst and that she would undoubtedly make a great entrepreneur.

Armed with this feeling of support and her own determination, Bel proceeds to learn more about starting a business, joins a professional businesswomen's club (more support), learns about government assistance and small business loans, and develops a business plan for starting her own computer service for small businesses.

These are her coping mechanisms. She doesn't wait for the right circumstances to come along, she applies her skills to the problem, creating the right circumstances to get herself out of the predicament. Since this is a success story, of course it has a happy ending. We find Bel two months later firmly established in her own business which she runs from her home. She is making more money, has no child-care problems and has more freedom and control over her life than before she was fired.

Knowing what could occur in a crisis situation enables you to understand better what might happen to you or to someone else who is involved. This knowledge will not prevent the crisis from happening, nor will it lessen its effects. It will, however, enable you to see that what you are going through is normal, and you will be able to recognize the phases in your own progression through the situation.

5. The 12 Common Factors in Crises

There are a number of elements that are common to most crises and crisis situations. The point to remember here is that experiencing a crisis is not an unusual event and that the emotions we feel and the ways in which we deal with a crisis are quite similar from one person to the next. Here are some of the things we know about crises.

1. Crises are expectable events in everyone's life.
2. Having a crisis is not a sign of abnormal behavior or mental illness.
3. There is no direct relationship between the event that may initiate a crisis and the development of a crisis. That is, what may precipitate a crisis for one person may not trouble another person. For example, losing one's job may be seen as a major problem and a true crisis for one person while other people may not care whether they lose their jobs, or they may have gone through this before and know how to handle the situation.
4. You decide whether the event will become a crisis or not. This is related to the point above. If the event itself doesn't necessarily cause the crisis, then what makes it or doesn't make it into a crisis? The answer is the perception of the person to whom it is happening. This is truly a case of "thinking makes it so." If you

think this is a dreadful situation and one you can't handle alone, it will be a crisis. If you take the attitude of, "So What. Who cares?" then it won't be a crisis. It's all up to you.

5. In order for an event to be viewed as a crisis, it must either involve a loss of something or the threat of a loss. Furthermore, the loss must be perceived as a serious matter. Losing your wallet when it has no money, credit cards or personal papers in it may be annoying, but it's not likely to be seen as a crisis. Losing it when it contains all of these valuable things makes it much more serious.

6. Not every resolution of a crisis is appropriate. That is, you may seem to solve a crisis, but it may not be a good or a lasting resolution. Some resolutions even make the original crisis worse. Think of losing a job for example. If this is considered to be a crisis, then it would seem that merely getting another job would remedy the problem. However, if the person lost a job as a senior executive and then took a job flipping hamburgers in a fast food joint, the problem is likely not resolved at all since the person will not likely be happy with this solution.

7. When a crisis occurs, people often stop to re-examine their values. Here's a true story about how this works. Bob had his own small business in a large city but found that his son had allergies to some kind of pollution in that area. These were so severe that the child was hospitalized for weeks at a time. Bob also discovered that when he took his son to visit his parents in the country, the allergies disappeared. The crisis caused by his son's illness caused Bob and his wife to think about what was most important to them, their son's health or living and working in the city. You won't be surprised to learn that Bob moved his home, his business, and his family to the country.

8. When people are in a crisis situation, they are likely to accept help. By the very definition of a crisis it is a situation that one cannot handle on one's own. So it's not unusual to find that the person having the crisis will look for and accept help. However,

this often does *not* include the people closest to them. The people nearest and dearest to the person having the crisis may not be viewed as having the knowledge to help or understand, or they may be too emotionally involved to be able to help. This is not to say that significant others (the people who are closest and most important) are useless. Usually, they provide a strong support system and are key factors in the successful resolution of the problem.

9. People's reactions to a crisis vary and they vary in proportion to the perceived seriousness of the problem. We've already seen that people react in different ways to the same problem, but their reactions will vary in keeping with the degree of anxiety the problem causes. When there is high anxiety coupled with a lack of coping skills, the person may regress to a kind of basic instinct level of functioning. Let me give you an example. I remember a boyhood friend who answered his door to a man who had come to tell him that he had unfortunately run over his dog and killed it. Jim was about 12 at the time and while he knew how to get along with adults, the shock of the news sent him into a rage and he attacked the man. This kind of behaviour isn't restricted to children. How many people have you seen who fly into a rage when faced with a serious crisis?

10. A crisis never occurs in isolation. The situations surrounding the event may serve to prolong or worsen the problem. Think of a woman who suddenly becomes a widow. The crisis of losing a loved one is serious enough, but there are many other things that take place at the same time. There is the funeral to think about, financial losses, insurance concerns, perhaps a court case if it is an accidental death caused by someone else, decisions about where and how to live, etc. These are not part of the original crisis of the death, but they are associated factors that will affect how long it will take to get over the crisis.

11. The more crises you have experienced and coped with success-fully, the more likely it is that you will be successful in new

crisis situations. This is really just common sense, isn't it? If you have led a charmed life and have never had to deal with any kind of adversity or difficulty, you will be quite unprepared to handle a problem. On the other hand, if you have coped well in a variety of situations, you must have learned how to handle problems and will be able to transfer that knowledge to new and different situations. The key here is in having different experiences and in developing a variety of coping skills that work and can be applied to other events. It's a little like strengthening steel. The more you have been through, the stronger you will become. Of course, carried to extremes, even steel will break under excessive pressure.

How well you cope depends in part on the number of coping skills you have developed or can learn. If the only coping skill you know to get your way is to throw a temper tantrum, you had better watch out. This may have worked when you were 2 years old, but if you lie down on the floor and kick and scream when the teller informs you that your bank account is overdrawn, it won't work. Not only will you not get more money, it is highly likely that they'll take you away to a padded cell.

12. How can you tell when a crisis is truly over? This isn't as stupid a question as it may appear. Many people think they have solved a problem only to have it reappear or continue in some other form. Because people having a crisis are often confused, they frequently have trouble deciding when the problem has been completely resolved. A complete resolution can only happen when the person's goals have been achieved. Of course this means that they must be clear about what their final goals actually are. Sometimes, a crisis counsellor can help to clarify and set goals.

6. Ego Defenses and Coping Mechanisms

What are ego defenses and what are coping mechanisms? Both are used to protect us from the trials and tribulations of the world and both can be used appropriately and inappropriately. Let's start with **coping mechanisms.** These are the skills needed to cope satisfactorily in our society. They include knowing how to handle your anger, get along with people, think through problems, find and use help, and a variety of other things that are needed in our everyday life at times of crisis. Coping mechanisms have to be learned.

Defense mechanisms, sometimes referred to as ego defenses, are unconscious tools that we use to protect and insulate ourselves from the realities of living. We do not consciously decide to use them and may not even realize that we are doing so. I want to deal with these two terms, defense mechanisms and ego defenses, because it is easy to get them confused and they tend to be used interchangeably in popular usage. Both can be used to cope with a problem, but one (coping skills) will involve an active, conscious action, while the other (ego defenses) is an unconscious response. Perhaps an example will help clarify the difference. Larry is troubled by a problem he is having with his boss at work. Over the weekend, he consciously tries to put the problem out of his mind and not to think about it. This is an example of a conscious coping mechanism. It is not denial, which is an unconscious ego defense.

A neurotic is a man who builds a castle in the air. A psychotic is the man who lives in it. A psychiatrist is the man who collects the rent.

—Jerome Lawrence

Here are six ways to tell what is an ego defense and what is a coping mechanism.

1. An ego defense is rigid and compelled. Coping skills are flexible and involve choice.

2. Ego defenses are based on internalized functions based on the unconscious past. Coping mechanisms deal with the present and the future.

3. Ego defenses are used to distort the present. Coping mechanisms are used to deal with the realities of the present.

4. Ego defenses are unconscious and involve primary thought processes. Coping mechanisms are conscious and involve secondary level thinking processes having to do with problem solving.

5. Ego defenses operate as if it were possible to remove disturbing events and often involve a kind of magical thinking. Coping mechanisms deal with issues realistically.

6. Ego defenses depend on subterfuge and indirection. Coping mechanisms involve an ordered, open attack on the issues.

7. *The Major Ego Defense Mechanisms*

There are many lists of ego defenses and each year my colleagues and I review them with our students. Being able to list them is one thing. Understanding them is another, and I have found that the best way to accomplish this is to use an example so that you can see how to apply the theory. Here, then are Anna Freud's original listing of ego defenses plus some others that you will find useful.

Repression

This is the unconscious exclusion of thoughts. There are many examples of this, but one that was made into a movie involved a woman who had repressed the knowledge that her father had murdered a playmate in front of her. Years later, the woman suddenly recalled the event and her father was tried and convicted of the crime.

Reaction Formation

This also involves the unconscious effort to keep unwanted thoughts out of the consciousness. However, it differs from repression in that a person may consciously act in a way that is the opposite to the way they truly feel. An example would be that of a woman who cannot admit that she is extremely angry with her husband and consciously tries to be very loving towards him.

Projection

This is often called delusional projection. In this situation, a person attributes his own unacceptable thoughts and feelings to other people. For example, a man who has a strong sexual desire for the opposite sex may say that all women are interested in him only for his body.

Isolation

This defense is used to isolate or insulate people from their emotions. It usually involves not making the connection between an event and one's thoughts or feelings about it. An example would be a man who is unable to show or deal with his feelings concerning the death of his son. Yet he becomes very upset when reading books where children die.

Undoing

This is an attempt to erase an event or act that makes a person guilty. Parents who have lost their tempers with their children and spanked or punished them severely may try to undo the event by being especially nice to their children the next day.

Regression

This involves the return to an earlier type of behaviour. I remember seeing this happen when a group of first grade children were put under extreme pressure to learn to read. They did so, but most of the class regressed to bedwetting and thumbsucking.

Sublimation

This is a mature or good defense mechanism since it involves converting a socially objectionable impulse into a socially acceptable one. An example would be a very competitive, aggressive person who channels these drives into athletics.

Intellectualization

This involves keeping objectionable impulses away by thinking about them rather than acting on them. It is a bit like isolation. People who use this defense mechanism may appear very learned and can talk apparently unemotionally at great length without ever becoming emotionally involved. They never seem to have deep feelings about the things they talk about.

Rationalization

This is the use of convincing reasons to excuse or explain certain feelings, ideas, or actions. It often involves making excuses for failures. The best known example of this is the Aesop fable of the fox and the grapes. The story is that a fox sees some sweet, juicy grapes on an overhead vine and tries to leap up to get them. However, no matter how hard he tries, he fails. As he stalks off in disgust he says, "They were probably sour anyway." This popularized the phrase "sour grapes" which you now know is nothing less than rationalization.

Displacement

This is another defense mechanism we see quite often. This encompasses the shifting of feelings about somebody onto another person. Usually we transfer our feelings onto someone to someone subordinate or weaker than the person who caused the feelings. An example would be a woman who has had a terrible day at the office. Her boss yelled at her, her computer stopped working, and on the way home, she had a flat tire. She displaces all this anger and frustration when she finally arrives home by kicking the cat and refusing to speak to her family.

Denial

This is a simple one. It has to do with the non-acceptance of reality. Remember that this is unconscious. An example would be a person who denies that something has happened because they can't bear to think about it right now. We all use this to some degree, but it usually doesn't last very long. When it is used too long, it can interfere with normal functioning. I know of an example in which a man got fired, but kept turning up at the office for several days after his termination. No one had the nerve to confront him and force him to see reality, but fortunately, he stopped denying the event after about a week.

Distortion

This is adjusting reality to fit in with what one wishes were true. An example would be a very shy boy who yearns for a girl, but doesn't have the courage to speak to her. He tells his friends that, "She really loves me, but she doesn't want her mother to know about us, so she pretends to avoid me."

Compartmentalization

This is the tendency to keep separate thoughts or feelings that really ought to be considered together. However, if one brought the two conflicting ideas together, a serious problem would be uncovered. An example of this defense is the criminal acts of soldiers who excuse their actions by saying that they were only following orders and that they had no choice in the matter.

Fantasy

This is nothing more than escaping from reality by daydreaming. We all do this and it can be a healthy release for frustrations unless you have trouble separating fact from fiction. I probably don't have to give you an example of this one, but one of my favorites appeared in the film "9 To 5." If you remember the movie, three office workers who hated their boss fantasized about what they would like to do to him. In the movie, they actually got to do it, but for most of us, these things remain fantasies.

8. How to be Psychologically Hardy

Have you ever wondered why some people seem to thrive while living fast paced, stressful lives while others who don't have nearly as much going on, can't cope with even a little bit of stress? What is the secret of success? Can anyone learn how to be less prone to the effects of stress? There really isn't any secret, but we have discovered that there are three major factors that enable some people to handle stress better than others. Two University of Chicago researchers, Kobasa and Maddi, found that stress resistant people all had three particular attitudes towards life. These psychologically hardy people, they said, were open to change, had a feeling of involvement and commitment to whatever they were doing, and felt that they had control over their lives and the events that happened to them. In other words, these people had similar attitudes towards life that enabled them to cope with it effectively. This is somewhat similar to the point I made earlier about crisis and the fact that whether one has a crisis or not depends on your attitude towards the event. Let's take each of these and see just what is involved.

1. Challenge—In psychological terminology, this refers to viewing change as an opportunity rather than a problem. People who rate highly on measures of challenge agree with statements such as, "A satisfying life is a series of problems; when one is solved, one moves on to the next problem." Obviously, people who think like this not only expect to encounter problems, they recognize that as one is solved, another appears.

What's more, they feel that this is the way it is supposed to be and that this is what makes a life satisfying.

2. Commitment—This refers to becoming absorbed and interested in the events and activities in which one is involved. It is the opposite of being alienated by the activities and things one must do. The issue here is that this high degree of commitment isn't restricted to just the things that one *likes* to do. It also applies to anything that one is doing. These people engage life and disagree with such statements as, "Most of life is wasted in meaningless activity."

3. Control—This has to do with the degree of control you feel that you have over your life; what is happening to you and your involvement in tasks. It is the opposite of feeling powerless. People who feel in control do *not* agree with such statements as, "No matter how hard you work, you never seem to reach your goals," or, "This world is run by a few people in power and there's nothing the little guy can do about it."

These three C's—Challenge, Commitment and Control seem to have a direct relationship to peoples' satisfaction with life and their physical health. These psychologically hardy folks have fewer illnesses even than people who have lower scores on tests that measure stress. What's more when they are under stress, they are more likely to transform the stressful events so that they reduce the stress. On the other hand, people who are not stress resistant use avoidance tactics to counteract the stressors. The latter group distract themselves by watching TV, drinking, socializing, taking tranquilizers, sleeping, and doing things that fail to have any effect on the stressors.

We've discovered that there are a few other factors that effect how resistant people are to stress. Your psychological disposition, personality, early childhood experiences, and social resources all have an impact. One of the most interesting ones is the role of social supports. People who have a family, friends, colleagues, and a wide social network that they can call on in time of troubles are less likely to succumb to a stress related illness. This shouldn't be surprising, since it is quite in keeping with what we know about the importance of support systems in crisis situations. The value of these support systems was clearly demonstrated in one study which investigated the development of heart attacks in high risk men who had elevated levels of stress and cholesterol together with electrocardiogram abnormalities. The one factor that proved to have more power to prevent a heart attack than any other was the men's answers to the question, "Does your wife show you her love?" A loving home relationship reduced the incidence of heart attack by 50% in this group of 10,000 subjects.

Knowledge and intelligence are also resources that can affect how resistant a person is to stress. This is because these allow people to see different ways to deal with a problem and to choose from alternatives. You can see how this is related to the idea of having a variety of coping skills available when facing a problem. A strong self-confidence is another important factor. People who believe in themselves and their abilities are better able to handle stress than those who are tied up in self doubt. In the final analysis, it comes down to the same factors we examined in the section on coping. Your attitude is probably the single most important element. How you choose to view the situation will set the tone for what happens after that. If you have a support system, take control, are open to change, and apply yourself to the problem, you too can be psychologically hardy.

9. Crisis Intervention: What It Is and How to Do It

Crisis intervention is simply the process of helping someone through a crisis. We are all called upon to perform this service from time to time. We may help a child handle a social problem with playmates, or comfort a friend who has lost a parent, or support a colleague who is going through a divorce. Anyone can be involved in crisis intervention, however, there are professionals who are specially trained to do this work and there is a growing body of knowledge about how to do it. Before turning to how to do it, let's see how crisis intervention differs from two other forms of helping—psychoanalysis and psychotherapy. In psychoanalysis, the analyst is a specially trained medical practitioner who helps the client focus on the past in an attempt to uncover the root causes of problems. The analyst does not take an active role in directing the clients' behaviours, but tries to lead them to a better understanding of themselves. This may take months or years.

A psychotherapist is also specially educated and may or may not be part of the trained medical profession. These professionals are only interested in the past as it relates to the present situation and are somewhat less passive in their approach. They may gently move their clients to a better understanding of their problem and may suggest strategies for dealing with them. A psychotherapist usually works with a client for a period of several weeks.

A crisis counsellor can be anyone, but in the professional sense of the word, it is a person who has acquired some kind of knowledge and training in counselling, psychology, and handling crises. These people are interested only in the present and focus their attention on the immediate problem that is facing the client. Their goal is to return the person to a normal level of functioning as soon as possible and to do this, they may be very directive. They may involve themselves in the client's problem, suggest appropriate courses of action, arrange help from other people and counsel the client's family and other support system members. The focus is on immediate help for this particular situation. Since the crisis counsellor is not prepared to engage the client in long term psychological counselling, these sessions usually extend over a period of a few days or weeks.

There are several crisis intervention models which set forth the steps that one can take to assist a person in crisis. Regardless of the number of steps or the exact sequence, the common elements are as follows:

Steps in the Crisis Model

1. Identify the major problem
2. Examine feelings
3. Provide support
4. Set goals
5. Examine solutions
6. Decide on a course of action
7. Provide follow-up

It is essential that the counsellor do a proper diagnosis of the situation and determine the major problem and it's causes. Often a client will have many, inter-related problems, but there is usually *one* that needs to be solved immediately. For example, people might come for counselling because they lost their job, are in financial trouble, are not getting along with their spouse, and are drinking too much. Which problem needs attention first? If the family is in danger of losing their home because they can't pay the rent, then this is the place to start since it is the most serious at this moment. Feelings tend to run high in crisis situations and both the persons experiencing the crisis and those around them may be angry, resentful, confused, anxious, or guilty. Often they don't understand their feelings nor the feelings of the other people involved. It is important to get these feelings out into the open and begin the process of communication with everyone who is concerned.

This leads naturally into helping the person establish a working support system. Often this will be the people closest to them, but on occasion, it will require the counsellor to put the client in touch with an external support group or other professionals. Before deciding on what to do, it is important to have a clear set of goals in mind. You will recall that goal setting is essential so that you will know when the crisis is over. After you have accomplished this, you can move on to help the person consider the most appropriate solutions. This is where the counsellor usually has to be very directive and offer specific solutions that will work. After all, if the people in crisis knew what to do, they wouldn't be there in the first place. So even if the solution seems painfully obvious to the counsellor, he or she must present it to the client and get their commitment to it. The next step is to help the client implement the actions and finally, there is usually a follow-up step to make sure that the crisis has been resolved.

10. Where to Get More Information

Aquilera, D. C., and J. M. Messick. *Crisis Intervention: Theory and Methodology.* (4th ed.). St. Louis: C. V. Mosby. 1982.

Brickman, P., V. C. Rabinowitz, J. Karuza, D. Coates, E. Cohn, and L. Kidder. "Models of Helping and Coping." *American Psychologist.* 1982. *37.* p. 203–212.

Cousins, N. "Anatomy of an Illness." *The New England Journal of Medicine,* 1976. *295.* p. 1458–1463.

Gilliland, B. E., and R. K. James. *Crisis Intervention Strategies.* (2nd ed.) Brooks/Cole, Pacific Grove CA. 1993.

Hopson, Barrie. "Transition: Understanding and Managing Personal Change." *Psychology for Social Workers* Martin Herbert (Editor) London: MacMillan Press, 1981, p. 141–165.

Kobasa, S. C. "Stressful Life Events, Personality, and Health. An inquiry into hardiness." *Personality and Social Psychology 37* Nov., 1979. p. 1–11.

Kobasa, S.C., S. R. Maddi, and S. Kahn. "Hardiness and Health: A Prospective Study." *Journal of Personality and Social Psychology. 42* Apr., 1982. p. 168–77.

Lazarus, R. S., and S. Folkman. *Stress, Appraisal, and Coping.* New York: Springer. 1984.

Lilfeld, S. W., Jr. "Coping Styles." *Journal of Human Stress. 6* June, 1980. p. 2–10.

Pines, M. "Psychological Hardiness: the role of challenge in health." *Psychology Today.* Nov., 1980. p. 34–44.

Wortman, C. B., and R. L. Silver. *Coping With Undesirable Life Events. Human Helplessness.* New York: Academic Press. 1980.

chapter 8

Transition, Change and the Future

It's the most unhappy people who
most fear change.

—Mignon McLaughlin

---

1. Introduction

This chapter deals with transitions and what happens to us during them; change and why it causes us stress; and the kinds of change we can expect in the future. As we look at the changes, I'll point out what impact they may have on us. One of the best ways to adjust to change is to prepare for it ahead of time. Of course this means that one must anticipate what is about to happen. This isn't as hard to do as you might imagine since many of the social changes that will happen in the future are already underway. All we have to do is be aware of them and think about the effects they will have on us. I'll conclude the chapter and the book with some practical suggestions for how to cope with change and reduce the stress it can cause.

2. Transitions

What are we talking about when we speak of transitions? What happens to people during transitions? *Transition*, as I'll be using it here, means a normal passage or change from one situation to

161

another. Levinson talks about transitions as bridges which cross a boundary between two periods of stability. For example, he says there is a transition period between early adulthood and middle adulthood. Golan thinks of a transition as a moving from one state of certainty to another with a period of uncertainty and change in between. Regardless of the way the term *transition* is defined, we find that there are certain common elements in all transitions. They mark a change that demands an adjustment in roles, responsibilities, and attitudes. The may come about because of one's age, the time in which one lives or because of something that has happened to a person. For example, a transition related to one's age might occur when a person reaches middle age and undergoes a transition to become what we call an elderly person. A transition triggered by the time in which one lives might involve the impact of computers and the need to learn how to use one in your daily work. An example of a transition brought on by a personal event might be a transition caused by the death of a spouse and suddenly the survivor becomes a widow or widower. Sometimes the person's age and the event are linked; for example, people get married and have children in early adulthood, and people retire in later adulthood.

Every transition involves change, adjustment, taking on new roles, a period of confusion and a time of discomfort and anxiety. Just consider the kind of role changes that may be required during a transition. There can be a change in a key role such as becoming a marriage partner. Sometimes we add new roles to the ones we already have, for example, when one becomes a parent as well as a spouse, or when you start taking care of aging parents as well as your children. Or you may exchange one role for another. This would be the case if you quit your job and went back to school and became a student. Some people may give up a role and not replace it with another. This would be the case with a widower who does not remarry.

No matter what kind of transition you experience, you will have to learn new roles, new ways of looking at life, and new skills. You can anticipate that there will be a period of adjustment and that this will probably make you feel uncomfortable. Just as we saw with dealing with a crisis, much of how you respond and adjust will depend on how you approach the transition. If you feel that it is unwelcome and a problem, this attitude will probably mean that it will become a major problem. However, if you approach it with the three C's of the psychologically hardy and accept it as a challenge, tackle it with commitment, and exercise some control over the process, you won't have a serious problem with the transition.

> *It is the nature of a man as he grows older . . . to protest against change, particularly change for the better.*
> —John Steinbeck

3. The Nature of Change

Like it or not, we are subject to change. Changes occur whether we want them to or not and the only choice we have is whether we wish to embrace them or to resist them. However, it helps if we get a perspective on change, how fast it is happening, and how people have coped with it in the past. "Ah well," you say. "Things are changing more now than they ever did in the past." Are you sure? Or is it just that we know more about change than we did in previous centuries. You have probably heard the statement that the only thing that is constant is change itself. But did you realize that it was Heraclitus who said this and that he lived in the 6th century B.C.? We assume that constant change is something that has only happened in the post industrial world, but every age has experienced major change. The difference today is that we are living longer and experience more changes over a longer lifespan. If we look at the relationship between the time it has taken to double our knowledge and the length of the human lifespan, we would see that at the time of ancient Rome, you would have had to live at least two lifetimes to experience a major social change. We are currently living two or three times longer than our ancient ancestors, so we have much more time to experience changes. But in the meantime, our total knowledge and technology have increased dramatically and we are able to effect more and larger changes in a shorter period of time. This coupled with the our instant knowledge of change makes us more sensitive to change so it *seems* that we are deluged with change.

Consider the speed at which information about anything, including change travels these days. The news of Nelson's victory at Trafalgar took six weeks to reach the new world in 1805 and even fifty years after the invention of the storage battery in 1798, few scientists in the world knew about it. Contrast that with the instant news that we get every hour. We don't have to wait for the news to arrive, or to find out about something by reading a newspaper. Today, events are broadcast as they happen no matter where they happen. People world wide watch sports events, wars and everything else as they occur.

In addition, our attitudes toward change have altered over the years. We have seen so much change that we have lost our fascination with it. We take change for granted and expect that it will happen. We assume that there will be another miracle drug invented, that it will be possible to visit the planets, that new products and new processes will make our lives better and we scarcely notice when these things take place. Couple this with the tendency to report only the bad, sensational news and you can understand why we either tend to disregard change or to focus on the negatives that accompany it. The old adage that good news is no news holds true. When things are going along as planned and good things result, this is seen as normal, boring, and uninteresting. Another factor that affects our views of change is our tendency to get upset at the minor changes that have an impact on us directly. A drop in the dollar on international money markets doesn't seem to affect most of us, but finding that our favorite snack food is no longer being produced sends us into a tizzy.

All of these things combine to contribute to a feeling that there is too much change. It is certainly true, as dozens of stress researchers have shown, that change causes stress and that too much stress can actually kill you. The problem is a combination of a great many changes taking place and the constant news we get about these changes even if they don't affect us. This contributes to a feeling that there is too much change. Alvin Toffler popularized this notion in his 1970 book *Future Shock* in which he pointed out that we often subject people to too much change over too short a time.

We can handle change. But to do so requires us to learn how to handle the stress that it causes and to try to anticipate and then control the changes that are likely to occur. Some of the points I've raised about dealing with a crisis and becoming stress resistant certainly apply here, and they will help you deal with change. It is also possible to anticipate what changes will occur and determine the impact that they will have on you. This is not a matter of crystal ball gazing and making the kinds of unsubstantiated predictions we read about in the tabloid press. Rather it is a growing, important area of respectable research based on identifying current trends and figuring out what will happen if they continue. I confess to being fascinated by this kind of information, and I am also convinced that anyone who hopes to be well adjusted must be able to anticipate the future and prepare to change with it.

4. Our Changing Demographics

Let me give you an example of a current trend and then direct your attention to its impacts. The demographics of North America are changing and we have reached the point where we have fewer young people and many more older people. This situation is a bit of a sleeping giant. Many people are quite unaware of what is happening and now it will effect them. Let's take a look at a few of the facts.

- At the turn of the century, fewer than 4% of North Americans were over the age of 65.
- It took 30 years for this group to double in size.
- By the late 1980s this group had reached 12% of the population and the time to double the size of the group was reduced to well under 30 years.
- The over 65 age group is growing twice as fast as the rest of the population.
- By the mid 1980s the number of people over 65 had surpassed the number of teenagers.
- The baby boomers are having fewer children than their parents, or having no children.
- We have become a middle-aged culture. The youth culture is now a minority.
- Most of the wealth in North America is held in the hands of middle-aged and older people.
- Around year 2011, the first of the baby boomers will be eligible for normal retirement. In less than 20 years after that, the social security system will be bankrupt.
- The elderly are living longer, are healthier, better educated, and more organized than ever before. They will become a powerful political force.

These facts coupled with the demands the elderly will create for housing, services, health care, travel, leisure activities, more accessible buildings, education, and a host of other things will result in major changes in our lifestyles, goods and services, and outlook on society. If you look around, you will begin to notice the impact of these trends everywhere. We have more older people modeling clothes, more products for older people, more older workers, more retired people, more special services for seniors, etc. The list goes on and on and it will continue to get bigger and more diverse. This is a significant social trend that is already well under way and one that will have impacts on everybody in our society.

5. Life In The Next Century

We have always tried to predict what will happen in the future, but what follows here about life in the next century is based on trends that already exist. The only possibility that these things won't happen lies in the occurrence of something to prevent the trends from continuing. Here, then, are some of the things we can expect within the next few years.

We will become a paperless society. Paper is well on the way to becoming a high priced, environmentally unfriendly, and scarce commodity. We currently use vast quantities of it and our usage is growing year by year. Every American man, woman, and child uses more than 700 pounds of paper a year and Canadians use 550 pounds. It takes great amounts of energy to produce paper and the production process creates serious pollution problems. Environmentalists and native groups are working to curtail logging operations, and it is likely that paper will become more expensive and less environmentally correct in the future.

A paperless society may sound like science fiction, but we are already moving in that direction. My generation grew up getting most of its information from the print media. The current generation gets most of its information from the electronic media. We have moved from being page turners to being channel flippers. The technology for doing without paper is already in place. I'm not writing this book on paper, but on my computer, and I can take my note book size computer anywhere, use it worldwide and send the words wherever I want to by pressing a button. When I finish the book, I'll be sending the manuscript (now an anachronistic term) to my publisher on a disk.

"But what about reading things?" you say. We'll read them on computer books. They are already on the market. They hold thousands of pages on CD ROM's and allow you to read the material on the screen, or you can listen to it via headphones. Some even allow you to view short video clips and to involve yourself in deciding how the story might end. Encyclopedias, books of knowledge, dictionaries, books of quotations, and a wide variety of other popular reference books already exist in electronic form for home use and of course our libraries are becoming more electronic every day. Couple this with the fact that everything that is printed now is prepared electronically first and then has to be converted to paper later, and you can see that moving to a paperless mode isn't as far fetched as it may appear.

Our cities will continue to expand, while at the same time, more and more people who can afford to, will want to live in the country. This trend is eating up more farmland, but our farming practices will change, and we will produce more, with fewer people. In 1940, 18% of the American workforce was required to feed the country. But by 1960 only 9% of the population was still farming and by the 1990s this had shrunk to 3%. In Canada, it takes only 4% and in both countries, we not only feed everyone, but produce surpluses.

The nature of our businesses is changing. We are moving from an industrialized world to a post-industrial, information society. The smokestack industries and traditional jobs and professions are disappearing but new businesses and careers are taking their places. For example, as we diminish fish stocks in the oceans, we are turning to fish farming. We can control the quality and sizes, and ensure that the product is safer for us to eat.

We're taking more control of things that we used to leave up to professionals. This even applies to medical concerns. There are already a variety of self diagnostic testing kits on the market for home use. These range from pregnancy tests to blood pressure devices. We also have software now that enables you to use your computer to diagnose your own ailments.

6. Some Changes That Are Happening Now

There is no doubt that we are living in a time of rapid change and that people are gradually becoming more aware of this and more interested in what is happening now and what is likely to occur in the future. There are a growing number of organizations, study groups, reports, books, and newsletters devoted to identifying trends and predicting where they will lead us. One of the most popular of these was the *Popcorn Report*. This book, written by a marketing expert, identified the trends that were taking place in the early 1990s and explained how they would affect us all. Popcorn's book is not considered to be a very academic piece of work by professional futurists, but the book shot to the top of the best seller lists, indicating just how interested we are in what lies ahead. Her predictions are certainly worthy of consideration and I've listed them here. All of them are already underway, so you might examine them to see how many apply to you.

1. Cocooning—This is the tendency to, as Popcorn put it, huddle in high tech caves. The idea is that we are exhausted by our daily work and feel safe and secure in our own homes, surrounded by our TVs, stereos, CD players, games, exercise machines, and other inventions that allow us to enjoy ourselves without venturing into the outside world.

2. The Fantasy Adventure—While we are escaping physically into our cocoons, we are also escaping emotionally into fantasies, but they must be safe ones. As a result, we have giant theme parks, adventure style hotels, adventure centres in malls, a new breed of adventure vacations involving organized bicycle tours, river rafting, photo safaris, etc.

3. Small Indulgences—This refers to the idea that we want to reward ourselves and the prevalent attitude that we all deserve the best. So, according to Popcorn, we splurge on things for ourselves and achieve instant gratification by pampering ourselves.

4. Egonomics—No, this isn't a misspelling of ergonomic or economics. It really is ergonomics and it refers to the drive to polish the ego. This trend is based on the drive for recognition, to be seen as a little different from anyone else, and the demand for customization in everything and individual attention from

everyone. This has given new meaning to the term "customer service" and every retailer knows that this is an essential part of today's business.

5. Cashing Out—This is one stop past the dropping out philosophy of the hippie generation. The Yuppies and Hippies are now middle- aged workers who have built careers. But according to Popcorn, they now want to cash in their careers, rat-race lifestyles, and live at a saner pace in a better place. This trend seems well established as evidenced by the urbanites who want country homes.

6. Down Aging—You've heard of this one before. It's nothing more than the refusal to be bound by older social attitudes towards what behaviours are appropriate for older people. Older people are healthier, wealthier, and more active than ever before. Consequently, they are doing things today that their parents would never have dreamed of attempting at their ages. Few, if any, 70-year-olds are sitting in rocking chairs waiting for death. They are much more likely to be touring the Yukon, visiting Disneyland, or enjoying a weekend at the Poconos.

7. Staying Alive—We are all more health conscious and working harder to stay alive longer. We have far more exercise clubs, home exercise equipment, and more emphasis on active participation in things than ever before. This is coupled with an increased interest in healthy diets, weight control, vitamin supplements, and examining the ingredients of everything we eat.

8. The Vigilante Consumer—Very simply put, this means that we are more demanding consumers of everything. Consumers are organized and can and do exert great pressure on merchants and manufacturers. This is different from the way it was a few decades ago when people simply took what was offered to them and seldom complained if they didn't like it. Today, if a

favourite TV show is cancelled, consumers can and do force its return. Consumers have formed groups and are acting as watch dogs on every conceivable product and service.

9. 99 Lives—This refers to the large number of choices we have these days for everything from clothes, to lifestyles, cars, foods, and everything else. Popcorn says that this vast array of opportunities has led to a "frenzy factor" in which we all try to do everything we possibly can. It's sort of a variation on the theme of "so many goals, so little time." Do you recognize yourself here? I certainly do.

10. S.O.S. or Save Our Society—Yes, Popcorn is a little cute with her terms, and this is one of the reasons why she isn't considered to be academic. Nevertheless, the idea is valid and it is certainly true that our society is much more concerned about environmental matters than ever before. We are all much more environmentally aware, and everyone has been touched by the development of new, environmentally friendly products and the creation of new laws governing what we can and cannot do to our environment.

All of these trends seems to be valid, real, and well in place. I see no reason to think that they won't continue, expand, and involve more and more people. The relevance of all of this is that if we are to cope with our changing world, we must be aware of what is happening and why it is occurring. Anticipation is an excellent stress reduction technique, and if we can foresee what is likely to occur, we can prepare ourselves for the changes that lie ahead.

7. Changes in the Workplace

Since work plays such an important part in our lives, identities, and self concepts, it is important to look at the trends in this area. Many of the changes are a result of three major shifts: the move from an industrial base to a post-industrial society, the impact of electronics and computerization, and the shift to a global economy. These factors have resulted in the following changes which are already affecting many of us.

- Unemployment and job shifts—Economists and futurists estimate that some 25 million industrial jobs will be lost world wide by the beginning of the 21st century. We simply do not need as many people to produce things.

- Changing job skills—Not only will people have to learn new skills to work at different kinds of jobs, we are reducing the skill requirements of traditional jobs. Clerks in stores no longer have to be able to count change or even punch the price into the cash register. The machine does it all. Secretaries don't have to know how to spell or punctuate; the computer does it for them. Graphic artists, designers, and architects no longer have to do things by hand; specialized computer programs do everything for them. Openings in some professions will diminish as computers take on more tasks.

- Multiple careers—Innovation coupled with the development of new opportunities and the disappearance of traditional jobs means that people will have many careers over their lifetime. This will require continual education and constant psychological adjustment as jobs become obsolete and new skills have to be learned.

- Globalization—As countries band together to form economic trading units, it will be easier to move from one place to another. This has already happened in Europe with the EEC and is now underway in North America involving Canada, the USA, and Mexico.

- More participation in decision making—People are better educated than they were in the past and less ready to accept decisions and orders from people they consider to be their equals. This has given rise to a demand for more participation in all forms of government and in all types of management. This is putting pressure on politicians and managers who must adjust and learn new ways to work with citizens and employees.

- More people, especially women, are starting their own businesses—The day when one could assume that a university education or preparation in a special field would automatically lead to a job are gone. So too is the idea of lifelong employment with a particular firm. Consequently, more and more people are starting their own businesses, often from their homes. Women in particular are starting businesses at an unprecedented rate and are doing so four times faster than men. Usually they are also more successful and stay in business longer. However, being your own boss, especially if you have a family puts a great strain on you and your home.

- Working from the home—We seem to be well on the way to a paperless office, but it may be that we will also have peopleless offices. Office space is expensive to rent or build and with modems, cellular phones, and notebook computers. It is no longer necessary to provide salespeople with a central office.

  Their offices are wherever they happen to be; home, car or a customer's back room. Many firms have already taken this step. Working at home or telecommuting have already become accepted practices for thousands, and this trend will continue to grow in popularity. The increase in affordable computerization, the ease of electronic communication anywhere in the world via modem or facsimile together with the resistance to hours of commuting time has meant that both companies and their employees are in favour of this innovation.

These are just some of the trends and some of the changes we can anticipate. What will they mean for us? What changes in our lives can we expect? Here is a list of *some* things to which we will have to adjust.

- More technological advances happening faster and faster.
- More older people, together with products and services for them creating new businesses and career opportunities.
- An increasing reliance on computers in all businesses and the home.
- A demand for more education for all jobs with computer skills being essential for most.
- A need to learn basic computer skills and to continually learn how to use new software applications.
- A move from the city to the country or a new country.
- More career changes and the necessity of learning new job skills each time you change positions.
- More personal involvement in democratic decision-making everywhere.
- Working from your home.
- Starting your own business or working with people who own their own businesses, often a home based one.

The time to relax is when you don't have time for it.

—Sydney J. Harris

---

8. How to Cope With Change and Stress

Everyone suffers from stress: we can't avoid it and we can't live without it. A popular misconception is that we ought to eliminate stress and all stressful conditions. Not only is this impossible, but it is entirely impractical since we must have some stress in our lives to provide stimulation. On the other hand, too much stress can literally kill us. The problem is to learn how to live with and manage our stress.

There is a proven relationship between stress and heart disease, ulcers, hypertension, and several other ailments. It has been estimated that:

- Premature employee deaths cost North American industry more than $25 billion a year—more that the total profits of the top five fortune 500 companies.

- More than $20 billion is lost each year because of management absence, hospitalization, and premature death.

- Approximately 35 million workdays and more than $9 billion in wages are lost each year because of heart-related diseases.

- Coronary disease has increased more than 500 percent in the past 50 years.

- One out of every five men will have a heart attack before the age of 60. As more women attain management positions, they too are suffering similar symptoms.

Managers and supervisors of all kinds are particularly susceptible to stress. Even if they aren't interested in prolonging their own lives, their companies are. The American Heart Association reports that the costs of recruiting replacements for managers who have suffered heart attacks is now more than $700 million a year. Given these facts and figures, it's no wonder that stress management has become a popular and an essential course for thousands of people.

In order to cope with stress, we must understand what it is, what it does to us, and how to recognize our own stress symptoms. Then, we should learn and apply stress management techniques suited to our jobs, lifestyles, and sources of stress. Stress is the result of the body's reaction to some kind of disturbance. Our bodies react to a stressful event just as those of our ancestors did when they were living in caves. Back then, when you suddenly met a saber-toothed tiger, you either bashed it with your club or ran like the devil in the opposite direction. Our bodies still respond in this manner and prepare us to either fight or to flee.

It's as if the mind shouts "battle stations!" Adrenaline is secreted, the heart speeds up, blood pressure rises, the lungs begin to pump harder, the muscles tense, perspiration increases and the digestive system begins to shut down in preparation for the emergency. If you either fight or flee, you use up all this extra energy by calling upon the resources you have prepared. However, in our society, there are often problems that we can neither fight nor flee from. Suppose, for example, you are called into the office of your boss, your professor, or some other authority figure to explain why you haven't performed to their expectations. Your body says, "This could be dangerous! We'd better get ready to fight or flee." But, in fact, you can do neither. This means that your body is getting ready but you have no way of reducing the effects. The result is what we know as stress symptoms.

Stress symptoms appear in many forms. If you frequently suffer from any of the following, your body may be signaling its reaction to a high stress load.

- depression
- fatigue
- irritability
- headaches
- back pains
- pounding heart
- insomnia
- too little or too much appetite
- upset stomach
- decrease in sexual appetite

There are other ways to determine whether you are under stress. One of the best is to take the Holmes-Rahe Stress Test. This is a scale which measures the number of life changes you have experienced in a one year period and matches those changes with the amount of stress they cause. Holmes and Rahe found that all change is stressful and that the more changes you experience, the more likely it is that you will suffer from a stress-related illness within the next two years.

There are many ways to reduce your stress level. You can learn how to do this from some of the excellent books found in any library, or if you are more comfortable learning with others, watch for stress management courses offered by local YMCA's, YWCA's, colleges and universities. If you can't get to one of these courses (because you are too busy and under too much stress), try to apply these remedies:

If you are angry, do something to release the anger. The worst thing you can do is to keep it bottled up. Exercise and competitive sports are good ways to release your emotions. I remember chopping a lot of wood when my sons made me mad. It seemed wiser than using the axe on them and it helped me cool down. If you can't exercise immediately, talk it out with someone.

Try to inoculate yourself against stress. Just as you can take a drug to ward off an infection, you can take measures to ward off or at least prepare for stress. You can do this by anticipating what will happen, what changes will have an impact on you and you may even want to set the horror floor and anticipate the worst case scenario. If you have already examined the worst that can happen, anything short of that seems easier to handle.

Get organized. Much of our stress comes from not managing our time and our affairs effectively. There are many books and courses on time management and you can learn something useful from every one.

Learn to slow down and give in occasionally. In addition to the frenzy factor that Popcorn talks about, there is another dangerous tendency; that of trying to do everything we can in the shortest possible time. This is called "hurry up sickness" and it is more a state of mind than something imposed on us from outside. My father had some useful sayings that I hated as a child, but they did put time in perspective. Whenever he did something that someone (usually my mother) thought wasn't quite good enough, he would say, "A blind man on a galloping horse will never notice." Or "A hundred years from now, who will care?" You can think up your own phrases to drive your colleagues mad, but the point is that we do it to ourselves and we can learn to slow down and not be so hard driving.

Finally, there is a little acronym using the work stress that sums it all up. It looks like this.

S—Social support: build people support for what you do

T—Time: get control of it

R—Relax: learn how to do this and plan for it

E—Exercise: do it on a regular basis

S—Salads: eat healthy foods and control your weight

S—Scotch or Sex: Either can be fun and enjoyable. The message here is be good to yourself and enjoy yourself with others.

9. Where to Go for More Information

Benson, H. *The Relaxation Response.* New York: Morrow. 1975.

Deutsch, R. E. "Tomorrow's Workforce." *Futurist* .Dec, 1985. p. 8–11.

Dychtwald, K., and J. Flowers. *Age Wave.* Los Angeles: Jeremy P. Tarcher, Inc. 1989.

Freedman, J. *Happy People: What Happiness is, Who has it, and Why.* New York: Harcourt, Brace, Jovanovich. 1978.

Golan, N. *Passing Through Transitions a Guide for Practitioners.* New York: Macmillian Pub. Co. 1981.

Lownethal, M. F., M. Thurnher, D. Chiriboga, et al. *Four Stages of Life: A Comparative Study of Women and Men Facing Transitions.* San Francisco: Jossey-Bass. 1977.

Naisbitt, J. *Megatrends.* New York: Warner Books. 1984.

Toffler, A. *Future Shock.* New York: Bantam Books. 1971.

Zwelling, M. "Futurama! Tomorrow, Brought to you Today!" *Harrowsmith.* Nov./Dec. *16*, 100. 1991.

Index